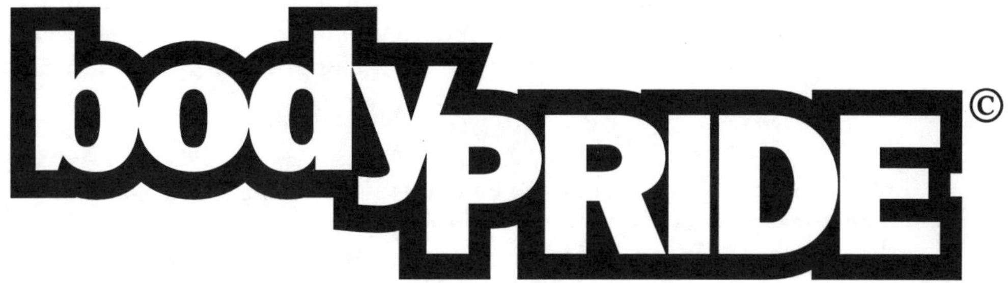

—AN ACTION PLAN FOR TEENS—

SEEKING SELF-ESTEEM AND BUILDING BETTER BODIES

Cynthia Stamper Graff,

Janet Eastman and Mark C. Smith

**Based on 25 years of medical success.*

[Another Lean for Life Book]

GRIFFIN PUBLISHING GROUP

This book is in no way intended to be a substitute for the medical advice of a personal physician. We advise and encourage the reader to consult with his/her physician before beginning this or any other weight management and/or exercise program. The authors and the publisher disclaim any liability or loss, personal or otherwise, resulting from the procedures in this book.

Publisher: Robert Howland
Director of Operations: Robin Howland
Managing Editor: Marjorie L. Marks
Book Design & Typeset: Michael Hendrickson & Ingrid H. Reese

10 9 8 7 6 5 4 3 2 1

ISBN 1-882180-81-X

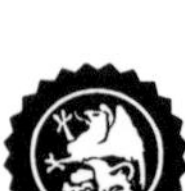

Griffin Publishing Group
544 Colorado Street
Glendale, California 91204
Telephone: (818) 244-1470

Manufactured in the United States of America

This book is dedicated

to all the people who strive

to make a difference in a teenager's life

and to the teens who let them.

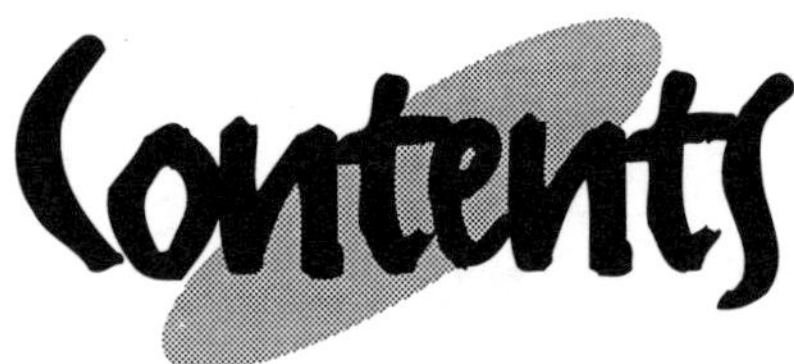

Contents

Introduction

Part One: FIGURING IT OUT

1. BRAVING IT • What's this all about? 3

2. WHAT'S THE PLAN? • What do you really want? 7

3. GETTING EXPLORATORY • The simple start up 13

4. GET MOVING • Exercise makes you happier 19

5. CHANGING YOUR HEAD • Good stuff about you 27

6. LOOK OUT! • Watch for body-image messages that hurt 35

7. BALANCING YOUR FOOD • Yes, three meals a day 41

8. ALL THOSE WORKING PARTS • Vitamins--you know you need 'em 49

9. SEEING IT HAPPEN • Your personal Daily Action Plan 51

Part Two: MESSING UP

10. TAKING A DIVE • Mark Lenzi springs back 59

11. SETBACKS • It's OK. You'll recover 61

12. EXCUSES, EXCUSES • Fight them with these five weapons 67

13. HARD TO IGNORE • Impulses are suggestions, not commands 69

14. SLOW-MOTION SUICIDE • The harsh facts about drinking, smoking, steroids, drugs and eating disorders 75

15. WIGGIN', STRESSIN', DEPRESSIN' • What puts you on edge? 85

Part Three: DROPPING POUNDAGE

16. SO YOU NEED TO LOSE • First, do the math 95

17. WHY DIETS ARE DRAGS • Avoiding that cranky, on-a-diet feeling 107

18. I'M WAITING • The real-food formula 113

19. NON-BETTY CROCKERS • Ingredients for meals and life 125

20. ROCKIN' • The importance of being a Mitochondriac®. 133

21. POWER THE SYSTEM • Revving up motivation 139

22. TOO FULL OR TOO EMPTY • Using food to hide 145

23. LET'S BE HONEST • You can blip and still bounce back 151

24. HELP IS HERE • Problem-solving is no longer a problem 157

25. LIFE LINES • Stuff that adds up to become you 163

26. FINAL D-DAY • Look how far you've come 169

27. CRANK IT UP • Adding foods to your meals 173

28. SET FOR LIFE • Stay fit forever 177

—THANKS—

Cynthia Stamper Graff is president and CEO of Lindora Medical Clinics, which has been providing safe, medically supervised weight-management programs since 1971.

Working on *bodyPRIDE* has been a life-enriching experience. It was a collaborative effort of the best kind with many people willingly giving their time, energy, insights and experience.

I'm grateful for Janet Eastman's wonderful idea to chronicle her son's progress while he went through the Lindora Medical Clinic's Lean for Life program. From his experience and her instinct, *bodyPRIDE* was born.

Mark Smith enlarged the scope of the project and brought it just the right voice as well as a quick wit and a reporter's eye for research. I couldn't ask for better partners.

Thanks a million to Ellen McGrath, Ph.D., who read the first few chapters for the integrity of the content and then encouraged us to complete it.

Alice Rubenstein, Ph.D., deserves special thanks for her caring concern and thoughtful insights that helped us present certain psychological concepts in a way they would be most easily understood.

Team Lindora once again provided an amazing source of support and enthusiasm. Special thanks to Olivia Moreno; Jan Hunter, R.N., and her daughter, Jennifer; Debbie Riley, L.V.N.; Carol Mulvey, L.V.N.; Meg Whittington, L.V.N.; Liz Castillo, L.V.N.; Brenda Long, R.N.; Kathy Sandstrom; Cathy Walker, R.N.; Cindy Alen; Kay Bennet; Keith McGuinnes and his children. Thanks to Lynn Nieto, N.P., and Joseph Risser, M.D., for their special supervision of the teens on the Lindora program. Thanks also to Peter Vash, M.D., for his conviction that we could make a difference in the lives of many teens. And to my father, Marshall Stamper, M.D., for his unwavering belief in the importance of early treatment for overweight adolescents. He taught me the importance of combining good mental habits with good nutritional habits in order to develop healthy lifetime behaviors.

I appreciate the confidence expressed by John Foreyt, Ph.D., when I asked him if he thought we had enough clinical experience with teens to be qualified to write this book. With 1,600 successful teens in our program, he assured me we did. I've learned a lot from John, especially the importance of "practicing" behaviors.

Thanks to Robin Howland, Bob Howland and Marjie Marks at Griffin Publishing. They believed in *bodyPRIDE* from the beginning. Thanks to Ingrid Herman Reese and Michael Hendrickson for their push at the end. Frank Groff's special energy is reflected in the cover concept as well as Bob Hodson's keen eye. Thanks also to Lance Huante and his design team at Piazzo.

And a special thanks to all the teens who gave us feedback, suggestions and participated in the photo sessions. *bodyPRIDE* contains a piece of all of you:

Aimee, 16; Anamique, 16; Ania, 14; Angelina, 16; Aaron, 12;
Chantelle, 16; David, 15; Eric, 14; Gena, 18+; Jennifer, 15; Jenny, 15;
Joanna, 14; John, 17; Kendy, 20; Larry, 16; Laura, 15;
another Laura, 16; Leanna, 15; Marissa, 15; Maurina, 15;
Natalie, 14; Patrick, 14; Ryan, 15; Sam, 16; Sean, 15;
and (last, alphabetically only) Tarin, 15.

Janet Eastman is a newspaper editor and mom to Eric, now 14.

I want to acknowledge my favorite writing partners, Cynthia and Mark; as well as Frank and Jerry; Valerie and Raisa; the California Scholastic Press Association Class of '96 and all the teens who graciously and outspokenly offered their thoughts on this book; and my family and friends who allowed me time to have fun.

Mark C. Smith is an award-winning writer and artist.

I'd like to thank Janet and Cynthia whose dedication to this book made it all possible. I'd also like to thank all the teens who gave their insight that helped us develop *bodyPRIDE.* Finally, I want to thank my friends and family for the joy and support over the years.

—INTRODUCTION—

HAVING THE POWER

Trying to explain this book is like trying to tell your friends what something tastes like. You say it's kind of like one thing, but not really. Finally, you just grin and tell them, "Try it. It's good."

bodyPRIDE was written for you. We want you to talk about it and come up with your own definition. Sure, we can let you know that this book helps you improve your self-esteem, do the right thing and feel good about your body, but that's only the starting point. You take it from there because it's custom-made to your taste. You're the one who develops the plan and then scarfs up the rewards. That's as far as we're going right now. But trust us; like we said, "Try it. It's good."

On the body image and exercise front, this book has elements based on 25 years of medical experience by doctors and nurses at a well-known medical clinic with 35 offices. But most of *bodyPRIDE* is about you rediscovering ways to make your life better.

Check it out for yourself.

INSPIRING TEENS WANT TO KNOW

Imagine you're standing in front of a million teens and they're hearing every word you say. What would you tell them? What's important for us to know?

Well, you have a place to express yourself—to communicate, contribute, link up. At your school, home, local library or maybe somewhere at your parents' work, there's a computer you can use. Click on **www.bodypride.com**, a free service of *bodyPRIDE* on the World Wide Web. Tell us what's good to know.

Also at the site you can read more about teens who are making a difference (add your story or your friend's to this list), as well as info on how to get involved, new discoveries in health and fitness, ever-changing trends and dialogs on what's really going on.

It's your world. Connect.

We'd also like to read about your progress. Progress? What progress you may ask. Your goals, dreams, wishes, aspirations. You know, what you're working on to make you YOU. Need more info? No prob. It's all in Part 1.

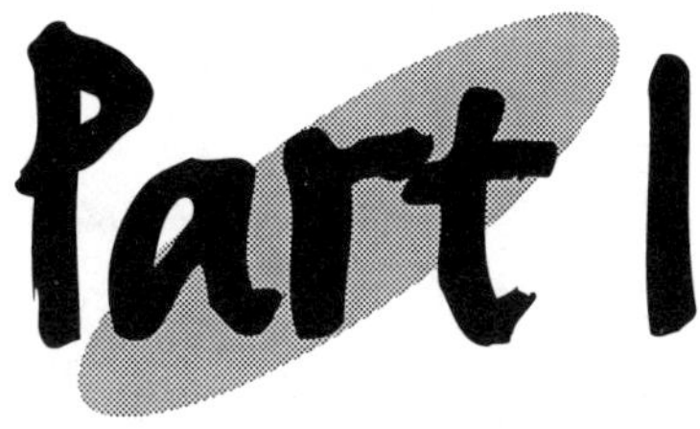

Part I

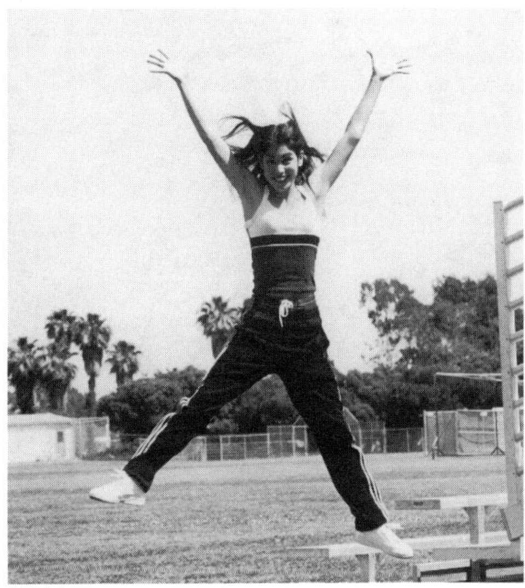

FIGURING IT OUT

In this section, you'll learn how to create a step-by-step plan for fulfilling your dreams—feeling good about your body, improving your grades, making a team, getting dates, improving relationships, dumping bad habits and enhancing self-esteem. You'll see how to change negative actions and thoughts into positive ones, and how to constantly measure and celebrate your progress with a personal Daily Action Plan.

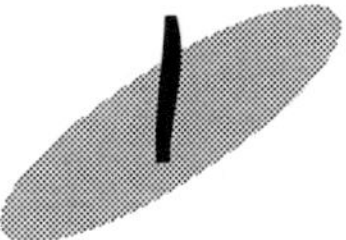

BRAVING IT

Everyone's been a teenager at least once. And it's a fine time. As long as the jerks stay out of your face, your friends are always around and that hot guy or girl is smiling back at you.

Ah, the perfect life. But being a teen isn't always smooth. There are times when things go wrong and nothing seems to work. You feel wrenched, stuck and maybe even helpless. Not such a great time.

But what can you do? If things aren't good in your life and there's something you want to change—no matter what it is—it's hard to know where to start. This book shows you how to get unstuck. *bodyPRIDE* is your workbook that helps you plot your strategy. It begins with you and how you feel about yourself.

MADE FOR YOU

Every day, parents get all worked up hearing about how teens are getting in trouble, hanging with the wrong crowd, feeling bummed about the way they look and searching in the wrong places for answers.

If you believe what you hear on TV, you'd think every teen but you is playing follow-the-leader directly to hell.

But we know it's not really like that. Sure, teens can stumble, but they also have the strength, intelligence and power to take control of their lives and their bodies.

This book is for you because you want to get the most out of everything: Make the team; make the grades; make a difference. Some of the teens you'll read about here have been teased by classmates because of their appearance. Some have been put down by the strongest cliques in the school. Others didn't have confidence in themselves to speak up and say what they were thinking, what was important to them.

But all have survived a struggle to change—mentally or physically—and they'll tell you how.

Start by remembering that you're the expert who knows more about you than anyone else. You know what motivates you. What makes sense to you.

"I can't stand those rah-rah, let's-do-it types who try to tell me I'll feel better if I do something they think is good for me. It's good to have help, but it'll be me that works it out in the end."

It's true. Nobody can do the work for you, but this book will do it with you. It'll help you pinpoint your dreams and then make them come true. You're writing it page by page, filling in the solutions and finding your way. Your DAP (that's just short for Daily Action Plan) will help you keep track of your progress. More about this later. So, what are you waiting for? Get busy.

MAURINA, 15, TALKING

"A lot of people think teens are lazy. They think my generation does things without thinking about what happens next. People think we can't make a commitment or stick to anything. It's unfair, but we have been labeled as losers.

"But I think our generation is a result of all the generations before us. And for the last few generations, the structure of the family has been hit hard. Our generation has to deal with the consequences. The concept of a family with two parents and brothers and sisters rarely exists anymore.

"I'm lucky because I can tell my parents most things. I don't talk to them about guys, but basically they know what's going on in my life. But some of my friends and a lot of kids feel distant from their families. It used to be that people would rely on their family first and their friends were outsiders. But now teens seem to be more loyal to their friends.

"The people I hang out with try to help out if one of us is in trouble, but what if your friends can't handle it? A 15-year-old can't give you the same advice that a parent can.

"To have a completely different life outside your family is too much distance. If they know something is going on, it won't be as big a deal to tell them if it gets out of control.

"As I get older, things get more complicated. I'm planning to go to college far away, and if I'm close to my family now, I'll be more likely to keep in touch with them as I get older and move away."

TAKE A CHANCE

Let's take a look at your universe. You know exactly where you sit, right? In the center, that's where. And, of course, there are people who orbit your universe—your friends and close family members (if you feel like it, get goofy and name a planet after them). Who else gets pulled by your gravity? Impacts your life? Someone from school, like a teen who's so into volunteer work? Someone in the community, like a politically active person? Someone at work?

These people thrive in your sunshine. They also influence you (but you knew that) and they help to define who you are. Some of these people are the ones you turn to when your life gets complicated.

Since you're in the center, you have the perfect vantage point to check everything out. From here, you can figure out which of these swirling forces are good for you and which ones you'd rather not keep in your gravity field.

LET'S THINK THIS ONE THROUGH

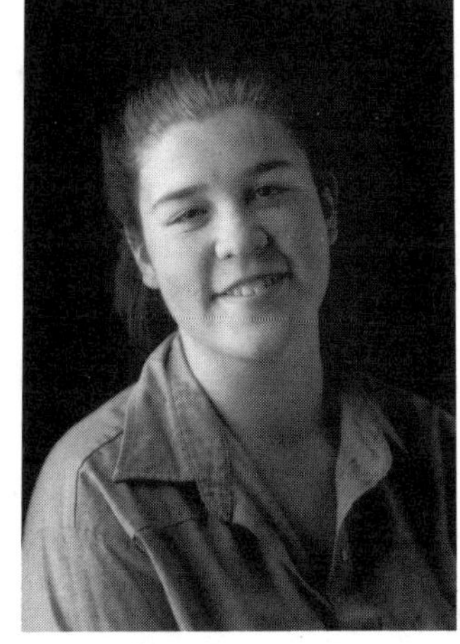

Of course there are things you can alter if you want to. How you feel about yourself. How you care for yourself. How you respond to outside forces. How you let others stamp their ideas on you. But before we get to those, let's look at the Rock.

You're in art class. In front of you is a chunk of rock. Your teacher has asked you to sculpt something out of it using only your hands.

Say what?

OK, this is a nice teacher. Instead of rock, you can use clay to sculpt your masterpiece but only after you admit that you can't change rock with your bare hands. (Sure some muscle head in the class may try it, but after going red-faced, he'll give up.)

The point of the Rock is to remind you that there are things about you that you can never change. Even if you joined the witness protection program and adopted a fake identity, they would stay the same.

Things like your bones. Whether they're small, medium or large, they won't change thickness over time. Bones are about as close to rock as you'll find. Your build—muscular (mesomorphic), round (endomorphic) or slender (ectomorphic)—will also be constant. Your size may change but your skeleton won't.

Then there's your height. You can't be stretched or shrunk once you're fully grown. Because of this, the length of your neck, arms, torso, feet and legs will pretty much stay the same, no matter what you do.

Other things about you that you can't change: Your skin type, hair texture, birthday, ancestry, genes (a swan adopted by a duck family could learn to quack but could never grow up to be anything other than a swan).

The point is if one of your friends doesn't like something that they can't change, be straight with them and say, "It's rock. Skip it."

WHERE'S CLAY WHEN YOU NEED IT?

Now that you know the Rock Law, here's the Clay Rule: There are some parts of you that you can mold. You have the power to shape your life. Others can give you ideas, opinions and guidance, but it's up to you.

Let's re-enter space for a nanosecond. In every great universe, there are good and not-so-good elements:

- **Saturn's** ring is dazzling but the planet's gassy.
- **Pluto** gets around a lot but it's too far away; real chilly out there.
- **Mercury** is nearby but it's super hot.

Now think of some examples from your universe, such as:

- **Mom** exercises often but doesn't get enough sleep.
- **Dad's** almost always on time but never has time for himself.
- **Sara's** a good student but she's down on herself.
- **My** friend ______________________________
- ______________________________
- ______________________________
- ______________________________
- ______________________________

Throughout this book, you'll read about ways to figure out what's good for you to keep and what you may want to toss out to shape the best you. You'll also see how you can mold the clay parts of you with a plan of action. Just turn the page.

2

WHAT'S THE PLAN?

"At first, you think up something that you really want, then you try to figure out how to get it."

We're not going to fake you out, straight talk is smart talk. Getting what you want means work. It takes planning. Imagine your life as a trip where you decide how far you want to go and how quickly you want to get there. You'll need to map out a plan.

Sometimes the trail seems like it goes on forever. You can only see far enough ahead to keep moving forward a foot at a time. But that's enough. With this book as your compass, you'll learn how to find your path, and if you get lost or detoured, you'll be able to find it again.

GET IT?

What do you want? *Really* want? Think hard and you can be honest (no one else has to know). What one thing can you change to make your life better, happier, healthier? Remember, this is your dream. Spend some serious time figuring it out.

Maybe you want to lose weight. Or be a better friend. Make loads and loads of money. Go to college. Be smoke- or drug-free. Create a safer place to live. Improve your grades. Cool your temper. Be a better driver. Learn ballet or another language or play a musical instrument. Maybe you want to go to Harvard or be the next star on MTV's "Singled Out." Or maybe you just want to feel better about yourself. The dreams can go on and on, but let's start with just one.

ERIC, 13, TALKING

"I wanted to go out for football because I'm tall and big and built for football, and it looked like fun. Every day during tryouts, I told myself that I was going to make it. I used to think differently. I had never tried out for a team before and I was never the kind of kid that other kids pick for teams because I was slow and I didn't really care. I knew I wasn't going to make it, so I didn't care.

"But this year I got it in my head that I could make it. My teacher told me that I should try out for football because I had the right shape, and I thought, `Yeah, I'm big. I could be a good lineman.' I worked hard to get in shape—swimming, running, exercising—and to build up my stamina and speed.

"On the first day of football tryouts, I was confident that I might make it. I did everything 100%. I listened to the coach. I ran really hard and I did bear crawls, then sprints. I was so tired but I kept going.

"My friend JP said, `I don't care if I don't make it.' Another kid didn't show up the second day of tryouts because he was too tired and he said he couldn't handle it. But I didn't want to give up. I don't talk like a loser to my friends so why would I talk to myself that way? On the second day, I gave more than 100% to show that I could push it really far.

"On the third day, I made the team. My two friends didn't because they gave up. I told my mom that I hit the jackpot and she said that it didn't just land at my feet but that I had worked really hard to make it happen. I was the jackpot."

WHAT IS IT?

"I want to feel good about the way I look."

C'mon, stop stalling. Write your dream right here:

____

____

Now, how do you make your dream come true? You get real. Think about something you need to do every day to inch closer to reaching your dream. What small steps do you need to take? Break it down. Do you need to take a class first to plug in to everything you'll need to know? Or can you ask an expert to clue you in? Would joining a club or a gym help?

"My best friend and I knew we had to lose weight and we did it by eating healthy every day. Step by step, pound by pound, we did it. our boyfriends always talk about how they've got bellies, but then they order two hamburgers and fries and go to sleep. And we always go, 'Hey, what's the plan, man?' "

To reach your goal, you have to be really specific. Say, if you want to play mean lead guitar in a band, you have to do more than just say, "Hmmm, to rock more than Van Halen I have to do some strumming." Go further and list the steps you need to take to get there, like these:

1. Save for a guitar.
2. Get a guitar (don't forget the guitar pick).
3. Call around and find someone who can teach me and not charge a lot of money because I don't have it. (Or maybe you could trade lessons: you teach them Spanish and they teach you how to play.)
4. Set up my first lesson.
5. Take my first lesson.
6. Practice what I learned.

etc. etc. etc. until finally:

999. Perform in front of a crowd of people; hear applause; sign record contract; get on the cover of Spin; go on world tour and meet tons of excellent people in excellent places.

"Some people are stubborn. They have to convince themselves that they can reach a goal. It's good to help them along by giving them compliments and encouragement; you know, don't get down on them but they have to do most of the work."

TAKE A CHANCE

Ready to put down the steps you need to realize your dream? Write them in the order you need to accomplish them (and be sure to leave room to add steps as you go):

____

____

____

____

____

____

____

____

Now the final question: When are you going to start?

____

Did you write NOW? Bing, right answer! If not, what are you waiting for? The year 2000 is creeping your way. Why not go with the plan NOW?

"I no longer see my future as something that will happen to me. I know the choices I make or don't make today will impact the quality of my life tomorrow."

DECIDE

What sets people who succeed in making their dreams real apart from those who don't? They DECIDE "I can," then get going on these six important things:

Discovering: How do you reach your dream? Discover bits and pieces of information that turn into "Aha!" moments: those times when you get it, when you say to yourself, "Now I understand how this works for me."

Enthusing: Pump up your feelings of excitement and energy. Studies of Olympic athletes and famous musicians show that a high level of interest keeps them kicking and at the top. Have you ever flunked a test in your favorite subject? Probably not. Figured out why? It was because you were excited and you made your enthusiasm work for you.

Controlling: Cravings and impulses are tough to fight. You know, like the way you go for the grab when someone dangles a candy bar in your face? Problem is, when you give in to impulses, you're caving your dreams. But hey, don't panic. Coming up in a few pages are some tricks to help you think before you leap (but first, there's more on DECIDE).

Imprinting: Good changes need to be permanent, like showering and brushing your teeth every morning (otherwise everybody would be holding their breath around you). Imprint the good changes and thoughts into your head. Make them automatic habits.

Disarming: Change isn't easy. It's sometimes uncomfortable and your brain or body may say, "No way." Don't kid yourself that everything is OK when it's not. Face the truth. Don't hide under a mountain of excuses or pretend the problem doesn't exist. Take a sledge hammer to excuses and denials that pop up every day, and keep building your dream.

Exercising: Physical exercise clears your head and makes you strong. If you're active, you have more energy and you can fight off stress and illness better. And here's a nice bonus: It looks good on you.

"I look for the right circumstances and if I can't find them, I make them."

Now you're almost ready to create the all-knowing, the all-mighty, the all-important Daily Action Plan. But first...

TAKE A CHANCE

Sit down with a stack of 3 x 5 index cards. On each card, write down one payoff or reward that will come from reaching your dream. Here are a few ideas to get you started:

- **I'll** feel proud of myself and know I accomplished something.
- **I'll** look sharper and feel healthier.
- **I'll** be able to buy new clothes.

"A reward to me is when I'm at a party and a band is playing and cute guys are looking and admiring me. And all the attention is on me and they're flirting."

Other rewards:

- **trips**
- **graduating** early
- **having** a day off and hanging out with friends
- **feeling** confident about asking someone out

It may take you a few days to write down all the perks you'll get for working toward your goal. You may be walking down the street or talking with a buddy when something just pops into your head. Take a second and write it down. Write all of them down.

When you're done, put them in order, with the most important one going on top. Move the cards around until you've figured out your top three. Copy these three onto three new 3 x 5 cards.

Keep one card in your purse or wallet. Put the second one some place where you'll see it every morning, like the bathroom mirror or your underwear drawer. Keep a third in a desk drawer or tape it to your closet.

The idea is to constantly remind yourself that you're getting close to getting your rewards. Without these reminders, you may lose sight of the prize.

In a couple of weeks, after you're deep into your plan, ask your friends and family if they've seen a change in you. You may be surprised by what they have noticed. These may be some payoffs that you hadn't thought about. If so, write these down as well. Make that list grow.

DO YOU HAVE IT?

It takes desire, decision, a plan of action and dedication to succeed. It's as easy as 1, 2, 3, 4....

1. set a plan
2. stick to it
3. chart your progress every day
4. celebrate your accomplishment

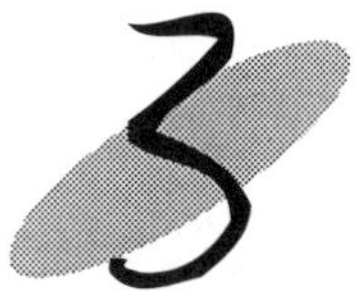

GETTING EXPLORATORY

Hot for an adventure? Maybe someplace where the jungle meets the beach and there's a surprise at every turn? Well, learning about yourself can be pretty exciting. Especially when it means you could take care of business and become a healthier you.

See, all this talk about improvement and change is really about a journey. And before you take off, you'll need to pack some basics—eating right and exercising. These may sound like old luggage to you, but they're a big deal. Hang in and you'll ace this. Skip out and you miss out. That's something nobody wants.

EAT

If you like the way your body looks, keep it looking sharp by giving it the fuel it needs with three balanced meals. Foods that are high in protein, such as egg whites, tuna, turkey breast and low-fat tofu, are a good start. Don't forget your fruits and vegetables. Experiment with new things. Surprise your family by cooking a healthy meal. That would wow them. You could make broccoli and watch your kid brother squirm.

"I soak skinless chicken breasts in fat-free Italian dressing and toss it on the barbecue grill."

Do you think you need to lose weight? Having a healthy body means that you're not too fat or too thin. Look at the chart on page 99 and see where you are. It shows a range of weights for girls and guys. There is no single weight for all girls who are 5-feet tall or all guys who are 5′8″ because bodies can be of different builds (that Rock thing again) and most teens are still growing vertically. If you're not sure if you're at a healthy weight, ask your doctor or the school nurse.

To lose weight, you'll still need to eat three smart meals a day. Zero-in on the menu on page 108. It's safe. Don't replace it with a crazy diet that says you should eat only pimiento olives or something weird like that. Those are fad diets. They won't help you lose or maintain your weight. In fact, stupid fad diets may do weird things to your body, like keep you from developing or make your hair thin and fall out. Why risk it?

And another thing (Knock, knock. You're still there, right?)—eat breakfast. Many overweight people skip the first meal of the day. Some busy people do, too, and picky people pass because they don't like "breakfast food," then they stuff themselves with junk food the rest of the day.

But guess what? Healthy people find that eating breakfast helps them control their appetite all day long. Grab control of your day from the moment you fall out of bed and sit down for breakfast. Do that and your day won't get away from you, not like that stray mutt you brought home when you were just a little dude or dudette.

Oh, by the way, studies show that teens who eat breakfast score higher on tests (math, science and all the rest). That's good, right?

TAKE A CHANCE

Write down everything you've eaten so far today. Sounds easy, right? Well, you may find that some things are easy to remember while others slip from your mind like soup through a fork. "What did I have for lunch? An octopus sandwich?"

Throughout this book you'll see this:

• BREAKFAST ....

....

Healthy snack ....

....

• LUNCH ....

....

Healthy snack ....

....

• DINNER ....

....

Occasional Dessert ....

Whenever you do, fill in what you remember eating.

"I dump Tabasco sauce on everything."

Now, back to more basics.

MARIA, 17, TALKING

"Change is hard but if you want what's best, you have to do it. I had to struggle at first to lose weight. It was hard because I was in school and I couldn't find good things to eat in the cafeteria until I really looked. And my family is not made up of healthy eaters. We're from South America and there are always fatty foods, traditional meats, rice, corn and breads on the table.

"I've lost 20 pounds so far and I already have more energy. I reward myself with clothes like short-sleeved cotton shirts and short walking shorts. I want to go shopping and start my senior year all trim.

"I work at a 99-cent store, which keeps me busy. I also work with a Catholic charity and make food for the homeless. It's such an experience. The first time I went, it was scary. Now it feels so good to help. I have discovered that everyone is so different. I love it.

"Everything depends on how committed you are and how seriously you take it. Go for your goal and don't let anyone stop you. Even when it's hard, you have to have control. You have to stay committed. Don't give up!"

DRINK

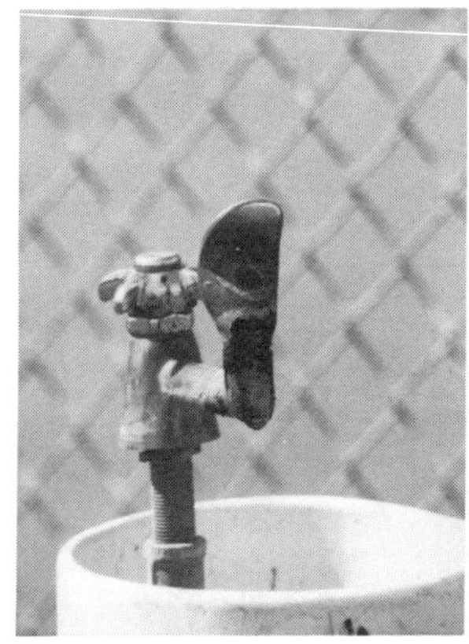

You'll need a big water container, maybe not Shaquille O'Neal-sized, but close. Say, 32 ounces or larger. This is because you'll be downing 64 ounces of water every day. Worried you'll need a wet suit? Don't, instead think about how good all that cool, liquid stuff is for you. You need that much water to quench your body, hydrate your skin, clear up your face (yep, it's going to help), clean your system, curb your appetite, reduce fluid retention, lubricate your joints and internal organs, and give you something nonpolluting (that's right, besides sodas) to hold in your hand.

Add a zippy little lemon to your water and the benefits multiply (lemon's a fruit, after all). If you don't like the citrus taste and find you're not drinking the water because of it, you know what to do—leave it out. The benefit of the lemon amounts to zero if you're not drinking enough $H_2 0$.

Here's a tip: Drink as much of the Big 64 ounces as you can in the morning. Fill up your internal reservoir early so you only have to sip a bit more during the rest of the day. If you're exercising, drink water before, during and after your workout to keep your performance level at high speed.

And another thing: Your water bottle should have some kind of design on it since you'll be toting it everywhere you go. Nothing wrong with looking good, but you already knew that.

Here's another symbol:

Every time you see this, fill in how much water you've guzzled so far that day.

WALK

Something else you'll need is a pedometer or step counter. It's like the odometer in a car that measures mileage, except this little gizmo counts up how much you're moving your body. It does all the math for you and sure beats going through the day counting steps in your head.

Clip it to your belt, waistband or shoe in the morning and try to tick off 10,000 steps every day. You'll be surprised you can do that. A day at an amusement park can crank you up into the 30,000 range. We can hear you now: "Mom, Dad! I'm going to Disney World!"

"The last day of school my friends and I went to Six Flags. I put the pedometer on the top of my shorts and everyone thought it was a pager."

Any movement you do counts as exercise on the pedometer, except shaking it around in your hand while the rest of you is scrunched down inside a bean bag in front of TV. But if you're dancing to music videos, that's another story.

"You can reprogram your pedometer to make it seem like you've done tons of exercise, but why cheat yourself?"

Great, another symbol:

Every time you see this, 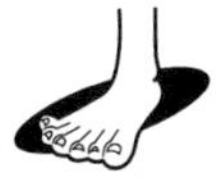 Guess what? Yes (you're so smart), you'll write in how many steps you've taken that day. Snap.

MEASURE

You will also need a bathroom scale to keep track of your weight, if you need to lose weight. People who don't weigh themselves are sometimes surprised that they packed on pounds in a few days. More on the weighing thing later, but get a preview of this:

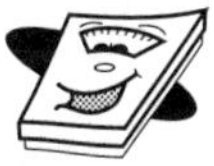

Don't head out to the store just yet to get your bathroom scale. If you're going to watch your weight, you'll also need a food scale. This gets you thinking about ounces, such as three leaves of lettuce equals 1/2 ounce. At first you'll be surprised how much things weigh, but after a while, you'll be able to eyeball a boneless, skinless piece of chicken and know it weighs 4 ounces (there's a mess of helpful hints on page 179). Then your scale can become another useless gadget that's laying around the kitchen like the microwaveable bacon tray.

No need to buy measuring cups and spoons—they're somewhere in your kitchen already, probably next to the cookie cutters shaped like bunnies. And you'll need to find a tape measure to mark your incredible shrinking body and to alert you if you've become overzealous and withered away to nothing.

The U.S. Food and Drug Administration has a free brochure called, "Should You Go On a Diet?" Write for a copy to the Consumer Information Center, Dept. 525C, Pueblo, Colorado 81009 or fax your request to 202-501-4281. Or you can download the information instantly at http://www.pueblo.gsa.gov. For more information, call 202-501-1794.

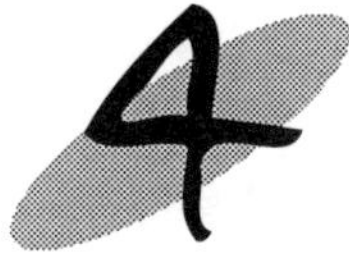

GET MOVING

"How do I want my life to be different?
I want to look better and I hope to get a girlfriend.
I want to be more physically active."

Exercise. What's in it for you?

Well, for starters, how do you think Brad Pitt and Liv Tyler got so fine? It didn't start with blanking-out with that video game or parking in front of the tube for days.

OK, those are big-bucks stars (look great, though, don't they?), so let's get back to reality. Besides making you look good in the long run, exercise has fast results, like cranking up your mood from worn-out to feel-good.

Exercise makes you smarter by increasing the number of blood vessels feeding your brain. That makes you more alert and a faster learner—you'll understand information in a snap and remember it longer. That means better grades with less work. Who could ask for more?

Well there's tons more. Exercise strengthens your immune system (you can fight illness a lot better). It also improves your strength, stamina, power, agility, flexibility, coordination, speed and ability to recover from or resist injury.

Thinking ahead, you can prevent some of the common problems of aging with exercise.

Right now, exercise helps your bones to grow at their top rate. It tones and firms and makes you more appealing to look at and touch. Oooh.

But that's not all.

It gives you something interesting to talk about ("Hey, guess what? I jogged for an hour yesterday," "Wait 'til you hear how much I bench-pressed today!"). It impresses people you're attracted to. Let's say that one again: it impresses people you're attracted to.

Moving on, exercise will help you sleep better and it brings an altered state of consciousness in which time flies and worries seem to go away. And don't forget that exercise helps you feel less stressed and less hungry and more graceful and more confident.

Exercise also converts body fat into lean muscle. That means you can eat more and burn calories faster. And you'll appear slimmer because muscles give shape and form to your body. It's the old riddle of what weighs more: a five-pound bag of sugar or a five-pound steak? Well, you know they're both five pounds, but check it out at the grocery store. Pick up a five-pound sack of sugar; it's soft and wobbly like body fat. Now go to the meat department and check out five pounds of beef. Solid, right? That's similar to your lean muscle mass. You'll want as much of that lean muscle mass as you can get.

The point has been made. So, c'mon now.

JUST DO IT!

A 1993 International Consensus Conference on Physical Activity and Adolescents recommended two guidelines for your activity level:

1. mild to moderate physical activity every day if possible as part of play, games, sports, work, transportation, recreation, physical education or planned exercise; and
2. moderate to vigorous exertion that makes you sweat and breathe hard three or more times a week in sessions that last 20 minutes or longer.

The bad news is only 50% of high school boys and 25% of girls get enough exercise. Girls exercise less as they get older—only 17% get enough of it in their senior year. Federal health officials have set a target for the year 2000 of having 75% of youths getting vigorous exercise three times a week.

Why don't you help lead the way?

YOUR CHOICE, FROM A TO Y

Acrobatics • aerobics • archery • badminton • baseball • basketball • bicycling • bobsledding • boccie • bowling • boxing • canoeing • catch • cheerleading • climbing • cricket • croquet • curling • dancing • discus • diving • fencing • field hockey • fishing • football • Frisbee • gliding • golf • gymnastics • hacky-sack • handball • hide-and-seek • hiking • hockey • hopscotch • horseback • riding • hurdling • ice hockey • ice skating • in-line skating • jai alai • judo • jumping • lacrosse • leapfrog • luging • martial arts • mountain biking • mountaineering • paddle tennis • parachuting • ping-pong • polo • post office (just kidding) • racquetball • roller hockey • roller skating • rowing • rugby • sailing • scuba diving • shot-put • shuffleboard • skiing • ski jumping • skin-diving • skydiving • sledding • snowmobiling • snorkeling • soccer • softball • squash • steeplechase • stickball • surfing • swimming • tennis • tether ball • tobogganing • track and field • tug of war • tumbling • volleyball • water polo • weightlifting • wrestling • Yachting.

The Department of Defense has a booklet called "Getting Fit Your Way" that lays out a 12-week exercise program that will get you started on being fit for life. For a copy, send $3.25 to the Consumer Information Center, Dept. 121C, Pueblo, Colorado 81009. For more information, call 202-501-1794.

FAVORITES

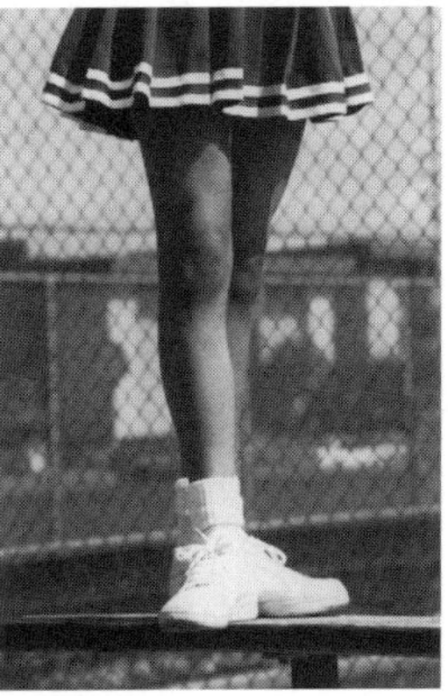

It's sometimes boring to exercise if you do it by yourself or if you pick an activity that you don't really like. So find a workout buddy (you can keep each other motivated that way) and a sport or routine you like. If you enjoy something, you're more likely to keep doing it.

The YMCA, YWCA, Boys' and Girls' Clubs, and parks and recreation departments offer inexpensive activities. Little League, Pop Warner football, soccer leagues and other sports groups teach lessons on how to play, win and lose, in addition to encouraging you to burn off energy. Sports give teens the power and confidence to compete, and a place to meet other teens.

BE GENTLE ON YOURSELF

The safest, most effective way to achieve and maintain good health is through moderate exercise every day. This means any continuous movement of your hips and knees that you do without becoming breathless. A big benefit to exercise is you'll increase the amount of mitochondria in your body.

Mito-what?

POP QUIZ

What are mitochondria?

1. Planets in a galaxy far, far away.
2. Dracula's daughters (the ones who like heavy metal).
3. Trillions of tiny, egg-shaped structures that dance in your cells and burn stored fat for fuel. Good guys every one. We like them.

BRAINS AND FEET

The easiest exercise is walking. You can't injure yourself—unless you trip over a cat on the path—and it's something you can do any time, any place, with pals or alone. You don't need to enroll in a fancy gym or use an expensive treadmill. Just brains and feet.

You can explore your neighborhood, the countryside or the inside of the mall (investigating the ice cream joints may not be a good idea). Go to the beach and surf, run, swim, play volleyball or toss a Frisbee. Or check out the waves on one end of the shore, then look way down the horizon and stroll a couple of miles to see how the waves are doing down there.

"The beach is my refuge when everything else goes wrong."

Itching to buy a few new CDs? Get one at one store, then buy another one at a store within walking distance. Want to visit a friend? Don't ask for a ride or power up the car. Strap on a step counter and, once you get there, ask your friend to walk with you. See how far both of you can go.

"I used to run but then I got burned out on it and my feet always stunk, my knees hurt and I just stopped. I don't have any problem walking."

The President's Council on Physical Fitness and Sports has a brochure called "Walking for Exercise and Pleasure." Send $1 to the Consumer Information Center, Dept. 125C, Pueblo, Colorado 81009 or you can download the information instantly at http://www.pueblo.gsa.gov. For more information, call 202-501-1794.

ZACHARY, 18, TALKING

"When I get the chance to talk to people younger than me, I pretty much tell them to get a part-time job when they're young and build up experience so it will be easier to get a full-time job when they're older. I'm really happy about my job. I'm a valet parker. Some weekends I work eight hours running to get cars all day long, but I can handle it. I wouldn't have even tried to get that job before when I was kind of lazy about exercise because I wouldn't have made it.

"I was motivated to get fit. I need to be able to get up and do a lot of running on my job. There are some slow periods, but when we have a convention at the hotel, we're working all the time. That's when I'm soaking up the money. I'm saving to get insurance for my car and to get some money to go to college.

"It's hard work but I love it. When you work, you want to be dedicated to it. It should be what you love to do. I like cars. The best part about my job as a valet are the nice cars we get to drive.

"When there's slow time, all of us start talking about how after we get experience and can go on to bigger and better jobs, what kind of car we'd like to buy. For me, it's a BMW 325, either cherry red or emerald green with leather interior, a sunroof and a CD playing alternative music. I can see myself with the window down and I'm halfway hanging out and my car is packed with at least four of my friends. That's what I'm working for. To make that dream come true.

"If you feel good about yourself, nothing can stop you."

EXERCISE RULES

1. It's how much and how often you do something that's important, not how many calories you're burning.
2. You need to make exercise a regular part of your life to stay healthy and maintain your healthy weight.
3. Don't exercise on an empty stomach or you may get lightheaded.
4. Don't torture yourself. Build up slowly (you're young, you've got time). Start with a few minutes a day and then increase it. Listen to your body, it'll help you figure out the right pace.
5. Be smart: Wear a helmet if you're biking, skating, Rollerblading or doing anything that might result in a crash. It's your head after all. Protect it. (P.S.: It's also the law.)
6. If it's really hot or smoggy outside, work out inside: Go to a gym, walk around the mall, you know the drill.

S-T-R-E-T-C-H

Before you work out, warm up your body by stretching it. You know how good that feels. Think about it. It's Saturday morning and you're in no hurry to get out of bed. And that feels so good. Before you get up, you spread your arms out, reaching with your hands out to both top corners of your bed and unfurling your legs toward the bottom of the bed, with your toes almost touching the end of the mattress. Ah, you feel ready to move through your day.

But what makes Saturday so special? You should give yourself time to stretch every day. Stretching will improve your posture, jump up your performance and increase your range of motion.

Here are a few limbering guidelines:

- **Five** to 10 minutes of flexing before exercising will prevent injuries and sore muscles. But before you stretch, warm up your cold muscles with an easy walk or a short bike ride.
- **Hey!** No bouncing. Stretch out slowly and hold that position for a few seconds, then release.
- **Your** breathing should be relaxed. Panting is for puppies.

THE FIRST STEP IS THE HARDEST

We promise, once you get going, you'll like it.

"It's not easy being fit. But it's worth it."

STICK IT OUT

There are ways to help you stick with your exercise plan:

- **Have** a backup plan. Don't say, "It's raining. Bummer. Can't run." Instead, be the first one you know to perfect in-house Olympic games (the solo or mixed-pairs push-up competition?). Or better yet, go to the gym and keep your family from going nuts when you start leaping over the furniture in "the living room high hurdles."
- **See** exercise as a way to get your thoughts together. "It's my time," says Heather, "when I can think about my day, what I did and what I want to do."
- **Entertain** yourself. Plug in your headset and listen to your favorite music, motivational tape, whale sounds or whatever. People who listen to something they enjoy have been shown to work out 25% longer than those who settle for the stuff piped into gyms.

"I exercise with my Walkman turned up as loud as it gets."

- **Reward** yourself. "After my second week of weightlifting, I splurged on a leather weight belt and my friend wrote my name across the back of it in really sharp letters," says Jesse. New equipment, clothes, CDs are all great. But food rewards are for babies, and when was the last time you had your diapers changed?
- **Expect** obstacles. Little aches and pains will come your way, but don't flip out or drop out. You may not get in all the workouts you planned, but did you make progress? Good deal. Pick up and keep moving forward.
- **Don't** get too gung-ho. Gentle exercise means you can do it for life. Torturous activity means you'll hate it and it may hurt you. "No Pain, No Gain" was an '80s thing. It's history.
- **Win** the argument with your slug side. You know, the part of you that says, "What does it matter if I skip just this once?" Let the active you always carry the day.

See this? It's your week.

	Monday	Tuesday	Wednesday	Thursday	Friday	Saturday	Sunday
8:00 a.m.							
9:00							
10:00							
11:00							
12:00 p.m.							
1:00							
2:00							
3:00							
4:00							
5:00							
6:00							
7:00							
8:00							
9:00							
10:00							

Block out all the time you're in school, sleeping, watching your favorite shows, talking with your friends, etc., etc., etc. See the blanks in the days? Those are your exercise windows. Use them. If you don't have any blanks, make some room. Remember "I can." Fill in the blanks with the exercises you'll do to get started!

Need more info? The American Academy of Pediatrics has a brochure "Better Health Through Fitness." You can have it for free if you send them a stamped envelope with your name and address on it to: Teen Fitness, Dept. C., American Academy of Pediatrics, P.O. Box 927, Elkgrove Village, Ill. 60009-0927 or call 847-228-5005.

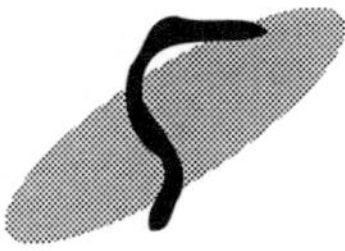

CHANGING YOUR HEAD

"Some girls see themselves as gangly or klutzy or fat when they're not. others used to be chubby then lost weight but still see themselves as heifers. Get on with life! Why go to all the trouble of getting healthy if you're not going to see yourself that way. Get it in your head that you're great! There's no reason to work hard to improve yourself if you're not going to enjoy it."

Your brain is a miracle, the wildest, coolest, most thrilling organ in your body. It makes the biggest computer with the zippiest processor seem as ancient as a tin lunch box. This wonderful machine, if you don't already know it, runs your body. It has a tremendous (big, really big) influence on everything about you. That can be good. But it also can be bad, depending on how you imagine yourself.

If you see yourself as scrawny or stupid or lazy, then that's how you'll think of yourself. Even if it's not true. There are lots of teens who may be just fine, and that's how others feel about them, but they cream themselves with negativity. What they don't get is that they can change how they feel by changing how they think. That may sound overly simple, even far-fetched (especially if you think lousy things about yourself), but you can count on it.

"If you want something to happen, to be healthy or get a date with someone special, picture it in your mind, in real good detail, and pretend that it has already happened and it will. I know it sounds New Age goofy, but it works."

Let this thought cruise through your head for a bit: Who's the toughest and meanest when it comes to you? OK, some grown-ups can be pretty hard on you, but you can be hard on yourself, too. You're the first to tell yourself, "I blew it" or "I'm never going to get what I want." We are too quick to call ourselves a failure, a loser, a bad person or ... you fill in the blank. But rarely do we give ourselves credit when things go well. Instead of accepting praise—from others or ourselves—we may say, "I was lucky" or "I won't be able to do that again."

Pull the plug. Push the off button. Just STOP! Those messages have a powerful impact on you.

Here's a way to look at it. If you were to use a keyboard to type a message, it would appear on your computer screen. You could type, "No one likes me" or "I'm ugly." And that's what your computer screen would show.

Or you could type, "I'm Happy" and "I Look Good" and "I Can Do It," and, of course, that's what will be up there on the screen.

Your brain is like a computer screen. What you put into it is what it will see. It just takes it in and acts on faith.

So, since you control the keyboard, why not type only good messages into your brain? Instead of thinking, "I'll never get a break," why not think, "Why not me? I deserve it as much as anyone else, especially if I work hard."

Another thing, these positive statements should focus on what you're doing rather than what you're *not* doing ("I'm eating salads" vs. "I'm not eating fried cheese"). They can also be statements about what you want ("I want to be strong"), instead of what you don't want ("I don't want to be the first kid who flunks the President's Council on Physical Fitness and Sports' sit-up test"). And you should make these statements as strong and as positive as you can ("I am succeeding") rather than wishy-washy ("I hope to succeed").

If a negative statement comes your way ("She'll laugh in my face"), instantly toss it out and replace it with a positive one ("She will go to the movies with me"). Sure, it may sound a bit out there at first, but saying it is the first step to making it come true.

There's no doubt that you may feel weird saying good stuff about yourself to yourself. You may think it sounds conceited, silly or untrue. But some brain experts say that if you say something often enough, it can help toward realizing it.

"I don't exactly talk to myself, saying, 'I'm better than him or her' or 'I'm too good for that.' I don't try to stick in my head that I'm the best person on earth...I'm just me. But I do say to myself, 'You're going to make it.' "

Let's first check out a negative example of how this works. A girl who wears a size 8 may think she's fat. She's not, but if she keeps saying to herself that she is, her brain will believe it. Then, when she looks in the mirror, she'll see an unrealistic picture of a "fat" person instead of the girl she really is. She'll always feel defeated.

A more positive example of this is when a bulky guy says, "I'm pumped and building muscle and looking great"—even when he's still flabby. He's working toward his fitness goal and there's a really good chance he'll feel so much better about himself that he'll work overtime to reach it.

Making positive statements to yourself doesn't give you license to fool yourself. You should always think positively about yourself, but don't ignore a problem. Recognize it, then find a way you can make improvements. But along the way, give yourself the encouragement to keep going. You can do it.

TAKE A CHANCE

Write down three positive things about you. Work on them until they feel right to you. Say them in your head or out loud when no one else is around.

1. I ______________________________
2. I ______________________________
3. I ______________________________

Here are some suggestions:

- "I feel good when I exercise."
- "I have energy and motivation."
- "I'm a problem solver."
- "I can handle any challenge."
- "I'm sticking to my plan."
- "I'm feeling safe, strong and comfortable."
- "I'm doing what's important to me."

HANG UP

Here's a good poster to put up in your room (suitable for cutting out and sticking up somewhere or tucking under your pillow):

> "I give myself permission to create and enjoy maximum health and happiness. I take responsibility for learning more about my body, my health and the many ways I can heal myself and improve every day of my life. I will surround myself with people, places and things I enjoy most. If I do this, I move toward accepting myself fully AS I AM...and loving myself without any conditions."

AIMEE, 16, TALKING

"You have to feel confident in yourself, to know that you're something, you're special, that you can do things. I've been a volunteer at a hospital for four years. I see that what I do makes a difference. You're a good person to the world. Figure out how you can show it.

"I wasn't always this strong. I was always putting myself down over everything. My mom has always had more confidence in me than other family members. If I feel down, I talk to someone who can help me push my esteem up, someone who isn't phony, but who tells the truth.

"It's always exciting when you haven't told anyone about a goal you're working on but they notice a change in you and say something nice about it. Then you know they're not just saying it but there's been an obvious change in you.

"You don't always succeed at a goal but you try again. I haven't cheated yet, but I may someday and I'll have to deal with it, get back up and start over.

"Today, I'm happy when I walk in places. I have confidence. That spills into other parts of my life. Believe in yourself and put yourself in the mode of doing something."

BUILDING YOU

Positive thoughts are super, but you can also create a scene in your mind to help you imagine what you want to achieve.

OK, OK, more far-fetched stuff. Is that what you're thinking?

Think of it this way. A builder looks at blueprints of a house to guide workers on where to put up walls, install windows and place doors.

Put yourself in the builder's shoes and imagine yourself raising the quality of your life in measured, positive ways. You have a mental blueprint of who you'd like to be and that's the plan you use. If you see yourself as fit, happy and successful—with all the rewards that go with that—you'll make choices that get you there.

Here are some examples of how to draw a positive mental blueprint. No, don't take a marking pen to your forehead, just close your eyes and imagine yourself as you want to be. In great detail. See yourself holding a report card with high grades. See yourself standing alongside someone you admire. See yourself crossing the finish line first. Many athletes picture themselves winning before they even compete; that's one of their first steps toward total preparation.

Still not convinced? Remember that time when you thought you'd screw up and you did? Maybe you pictured yourself missing the ball or failing a test or arriving after the bus was already chugging and blowing smoke down the street. You may have helped make it all happen because you told your brain that it would happen and your brain sent signals out to all corners of your body to make it happen.

Now flip it: Use this to your advantage. Picture yourself doing things right. The more detailed your mental image is, the more of a guide it will be. You'll find ways to make those changes come true. Anyway, you'll feel better about yourself, just because a good self-image leads to a good life. Watch what happens.

If things don't happen soon enough, don't get discouraged. You're that builder again, trying to find the obstacle that's getting in the way. It can help to ask yourself these questions:

1. "What do I think I'm supposed to be doing?"
2. "What does my mental blueprint say I'm supposed to be doing in this situation?"
3. "If my mental blueprint shows me not succeeding, how can I change it to make things better?"

TAKE A CHANCE

Think about your mental blueprint. What do you want? Why? What surrounds you? Who else is in the picture? How will your success enhance your life, health, appearance, self-esteem, relationships? Be honest. It's a blueprint of your future.

GET OUT YOUR CLUNKY BOOTS

If negative thoughts are sneaking into your head, stomp them with these tricks:

1. Listen to yourself. Be sensitive to your thoughts and feelings. To be successful, you need to learn different habits and skills. One of the most important skills is listening to yourself.
2. Replace negative thoughts and statements with positive ones. Make a game out of it. This doesn't mean to tell yourself you're looking forward to going to the gym when you don't feel comfortable with all the body-judging that goes on there. Instead, you can say something like, "I love the way my body and muscles feel after I exercise. I sleep better at night and have more energy during the day. And I feel better about myself because I know I'm making progress toward my goal." Or something that works for you.

   Maria doesn't always feel so great about working out, but she's developed a mindset that helps her. She likes to see her trips to the gym as "traveling." She brings her "passport" (gym card) and "suitcase" (gym bag), changes in "customs" (locker room) and says to her friends who ask her out to dinner, "Sorry, can't. I'm traveling." When she says that, it doesn't seem at all like she's losing out.
3. Accept praise. When you hear a compliment, don't discount it or ignore it. Look into that person's eyes and say, "Thanks." Period. Then let the thought dance in your head for awhile.

WHO HAS THE MIKE?

Have you ever seen that movie "Sybil"? You know, the one about the woman who suffered from multiple personalities talking in her head and trying to control her? It was sad. And crazy, right? Well, we don't mean to freak you out but everyone has different voices in their head. You too. Think about these voices:

Your Frightened Voice: "I'm afraid I'm not going to do this right."
Your Angry Voice: "I'm never allowed to do or say what I want!"
Your Hard-on-You Voice: "Don't even bother—you're not good enough."
Your Happy Voice: "Hey, let's do it! It'll be fun!"
Your Curious Voice: "I'll figure out a way to do this."
Your Loving Voice: "I'm awesome."
Your Confident Voice: "I can do it!"

Which voices of yours should have the microphone?

FINAL THOUGHTS ON THOUGHTS

Brena says, "It's really funny. One day I asked my three girlfriends who they thought was the prettiest girl they knew. Jennifer said Kirsty Hume because she's tall, a nice person and has long blond hair. I'm looking right at Jennifer and I thought, 'Crazy! That's exactly how I would describe Jennifer.' Then I asked Laura, and she said that girl from 'The Return of the Blue Lagoon,' because she's a singer and an actress and a supermodel and gorgeous with long, light brown hair, a tan and blue-green eyes. Laura has long, light brown hair. She's tan and has blue-green eyes! Then I asked Vanessa and she said Winona Ryder because she is herself and doesn't play lame people in movies, has rad boyfriends and is pretty but doesn't try to be. And that's Vanessa, perfectly, except she's not an actress. They all admired people who had the same traits and physical characteristics they do, but when I ask them if they think they are pretty, they say, No!"

"What's this all about?"

The answer: We've already said it but it bears repeating—we're harder on ourselves than we would ever think of being toward anyone else. Why not treat yourself better starting now.

CONFIDENCE IN ME

Does that new guy or girl in school really feel that at-ease with things, or is he or she faking confidence? Shsssh. Don't tell anyone but it really doesn't matter. In fact, acting confident can make you confident.

"Some say, 'Act as if until you feel it.'"

Need some quick ways you can show the world that you're in control? Try these:

1. See yourself as being perfectly composed. Before a scary event, close your eyes and think of something that makes you feel good about yourself, that creates a sense of well-being, like your favorite song or place to relax. Actors do this all the time.
2. Enter a room as if you own it. Walk in with your back straight, your head held high and an expression on your face that shows the world that you're in charge of your destiny.

   Studies show that people's first impression of you is based on how you enter a room. Those with long strides are seen as independent, open and happier than those who drag their feet.

   Think of it as owning—or temporarily renting—the space around you. Walk in as if you've just accomplished the impossible.
3. Pick a role model. Who do you know who's a natural-born schmoozer? Borrow qualities from them. Do they ask people questions to kick-start the conversation? Do they listen and react to what was said, rather than worrying what they'll have to say? You can do it. Everyone has the skills to be friendly.
4. Practice being bold. Confidence is a muscle that you need to work out every day. Talk to someone new every day.
5. Dress comfortably. It's hard to be relaxed when you're worried about your fussy clothes getting wrinkled. Wear what makes you feel good about yourself, what expresses the inside you.
6. Recognize your afraid signs—sweaty palms, hunched shoulders, that about-to-pass-out feeling. OK. Fine, you have these. We all do. Now relax. No one ever died of embarrassment. You can accept these things about yourself and go forward.
7. Be friendly. Everyone's waiting to be asked a question or get a shiny smile from someone else. Go first. You don't have to be as instantly entertaining as Cosmo Kramer or Rosie O'Donnell, just be friendly. Ask a question that requires more than a yes or no answer and then you're off to a fine start. Smile, gesture, lean forward, catch someone's eye, speak in a voice that's lively. Your actions will energize the encounter.
8. Joking about yourself is great with people who love you, but it may give a newcomer the wrong impression, like, "please pity me."
9. Say what you mean. Speak with conviction...and listen to the other side.
10. Let compliments sink it. When you hear someone say something nice about you, inscribe it into your long-term memory. Play it over and over again in your head. Don't let a reward fly away. You've earned it.

LOOK OUT!

"I want to be an inventor. I wish right now I could come up with something that blocked out the jokes kids make about me."

It's hard to be different, especially when you're young. Even the little things can make trouble. Eating something your grandmother used to make in the country she grew up in may cause others to sniff and say, "Gross."

Some girls just grow up faster, and they can be teased big-time for that. Slow-to-grow boys also feel the heat and are called names. A teen's nose may be large or a birthmark on their face may inspire cruel jokes. There's heavy, sometimes painful pressure to look like everyone else.

Even little kids can spot differences in other people's faces, height and body shape. And they point it out. Loudly. It happens as early as kindergarten.Who has control of what they look like in kindergarten?

"As little girls, bathing suits didn't scare us as they do now. We loved going to the pool to play in the water. What happened? Hormones and the opposite sex."

We're supposed to grow up and feel good about who we are, not just concentrate on what we look like. But that's not always the case. Just check out some of the messages that are out there and how they've changed from the Dark Ages to today:

- **[1950]** You know those stiff statues that stores use to show off their clothes? Well, mannequins used to be modeled after real live women. In the '50s, they were rounder and wider. But then manufacturers started making mannequins thinner and thinner, and now they fill out clothes about as well as a wire hanger does. How can we expect to fit a dress the way a dummy does? Better question, why would we compare ourselves to a dummy?

- **[1960]** Marilyn Monroe, whose platinum hair and curvy body have been copied by Madonna and Mira Sorvino, wore a size 12-14 in the '60s. When People magazine named its 50 Most Beautiful People in 1996, they listed all the women's dress sizes. Most were a teeny-weenie size 4. Who can compete with those figures? And why should we?
- **[1970]** Magazines read by teen girls in the '70s had 10 times more articles on nutrition and fitness than magazines today, which emphasize weight loss and personal appearance. Today's message is clear: lose weight (whether you need to or not) and become more attractive. That's dead wrong.
- **[1980]** Models' bodies have fewer curves now than they did in the '80s. Calvin Klein models' hip/waist ratio is smaller than previous years, making them look like pencils.

It's no wonder that a lot of girls feel pressure to emulate supermodels. Some obsess over it. They think about the shape and size of their body every minute. They feel ugly and self-conscious no matter how many compliments they get. They gaze in the mirror and see what no one else does: A big fat flaw.

Dr. Ellen McGrath calls these negative feelings of shame, contempt and disappointment "body image depression." In her book, "When Feeling Bad Is Good," she says too many of us "attempt to live up to impossible cultural standards of physical perfection, beauty, sex appeal, youth and fashion."

A survey of 12,000 high school students by the National Centers for Disease Control and Prevention found 50% of the girls interviewed were on diets even though only one out of every four of the dieting girls was actually overweight. Only 15% of high school guys said they have been on a diet.

It's pretty clear that girls get hit the hardest. Some grow up feeling that if they aren't beautiful, they aren't anything.

"I stand in front of my full-length mirror and wonder if I have cottage-cheese thighs. Is my stomach mushy and round like a jelly roll? Are my arms too jiggly and wiggly, waving gently as I say, 'Hi'? All my friends seem to have been bitten by this poisonous bug called self-doubt, and it's affecting me. I keep thinking, 'If she thinks she's fat, what does she think of me?' "

What if someone says brown eyes are nicer, but yours are blue? Thin's better than fat. Curly hair instead of straight, or is it straight hair instead of curly? Rich rather than poor. Hightops not low. CK jeans vs. that other brand.

Give it a rest! And give yourself a break.

"Every little girl dreams of being Barbie so she can capture Ken's heart and live happily ever after. We have this ideal figure in mind, but most of us don't grow into that."

You may want to trace your body roots. Maybe you have your Uncle Frank's chin. And it bugs you. OK. And how does Uncle Frank feel about it? Seems it's never bothered him, and in fact, he says, people have always seen him as a confident, take-charge guy because of his prominent chin (isn't it unfair how people assume you're one way because of the way you look?).

But maybe that chin can work to your advantage as well as it did for Uncle Frank. Or maybe you should just forget about it. That's probably the best way to handle something as hard-to-change as a chin. There are some givens you'll just have to accept. It's rock. Skip it.

Instead of being embarrassed and asking, "Why can't I be like the others?" figure out what you really want—better friends, higher grades, to play an instrument, get a job, finish a project, help someone. Then plan out how you'll do it. See yourself as a problem solver, not a victim.

If you want, try coming up with your own definition of what's healthy and attractive. Or think of people you admire and remind yourself that the world's greatest doers are valued and respected more for their character and courage than their physical perfection.

And if you know someone who is down because she doesn't look like someone on TV, clip a photograph of a ridiculously thin model or a plastic-surgeon junkie out of a magazine to show how extreme the so-called ideal has become. Or write your friend an encouraging letter or spend time with her doing something fun.

"It's really hard to not judge a book by its cover in our world. It's because a person's strongest sense seems to be sight and the first impression is made by looking at someone. Maybe some of us should wear little signs around our neck that say. 'I'm worth getting to know.' We all have to be willing to look at people a little differently."

Actress-model Tyra Banks tosses off the importance of looks this way: "Oh, when it comes to women looking at magazines, enjoy it and then put it down because it's all fantasy and a lot of it is fake. A lot of it is pins and tucks and nips and a lot of retouching, too. I hate it when women look at magazines and models, and get insecure. They don't know that if they were to see me standing naked with no makeup on and my hair not done, they would feel a lot more comfortable."

A REAL SIMPLE FACT

Skin's supposed to jiggle.

YOUR BODY'S NOT AT FAULT

Couples break up for a lot of reasons. Maybe you weren't nice to each other anymore. Or maybe the jokes you both kept making didn't get the other to laugh any longer. Maybe one of you met someone else.

Sure, there are a million reasons to break up with someone, but only one thing to remember: Your body is not to blame. Someone may say it is, but you know better.

Listen: Be happy with who you are. You don't need someone else to make you feel special.

"I'm comfortable with myself. I would like to be a little taller, but I'm enough. I'm a good person on the inside."

ONE GIRL'S LIST OF WHAT'S GREAT ABOUT GIRLS

"My favorite girlfriends are funny, nice, cool, entertaining, smart, kind, athletic and original. They're not conceited, trendy or lame. They're outgoing and considerate. They don't try to be someone they're not. They're good listeners and can keep a secret. They're not flirtatious. They're honest and always have something to talk about. They're understanding, loyal, open, supportive and not airheads."

ONE GIRL'S LIST OF WHAT'S GREAT ABOUT GUYS

"The best guys are soccer players! They're involved in school, like ASB officers. They know what's going on outside their home. They're not just TV watchers. They're smart. They aren't slackers who get bad grades or don't call. They just don't care what others think and they are true to themselves. They have nice smiles and eyes that stand out. They're not obsessive pigheads or sexist. They're funny, romantic, honest, different, polite, charming, respectful, faithful, trustworthy and understanding."

ONE GUY'S LIST OF WHAT'S GREAT ABOUT GUYS

"A good guy friend is someone who's comfortable to be around, who's not trying for social status and who will stay away from my girlfriend. He's cool and not judgmental. Someone you can say something stupid to and he will get it right away. He's friendly, open, smart, funny and likes sports. He's not annoying and he can't take offense. Someone who's artistic and shows it. He's honest, sincere and supportive. We share common interests. He's always there to help and is easy to talk to. You know you can do whatever when you're together."

ONE GUY'S LIST OF WHAT'S GREAT ABOUT GIRLS

"I like girls who are funny, smart, attractive, faithful and who smell good. They have confidence, energy, motivation, integrity, humility and compassion. They know exactly what to do to make you feel like your life is the greatest gift your parents gave you. They listen, put up with you and act mature but give you a break for being immature sometimes. They act naturally and are comfortable with themselves."

TUBE DAMAGE

Besides dishing out shallow messages that we should prize looks above everything else, TV can be hazardous to your health. You have control of the remote. Think about this before you turn on the set:

- **The** typical teen spends three hours watching TV every day. Is that you? If so, you should know that a University of California, Irvine study found that high blood cholesterol levels in 2- to 20-year-olds are directly tied to their heavy TV time.
- **Teens** are picking TV watching over action. If you're lucky enough to have exercise equipment (like a stationary bike) parked in front of a TV, that's great because you can work out while you watch.

But beware: you're also being exposed to junk-food commercials luring you into bad food habits. If you find yourself snacking—or thinking about it—more than you'd like to, turn off or unplug the set. You'll begin to notice that your mind is off food and onto something much more interesting.

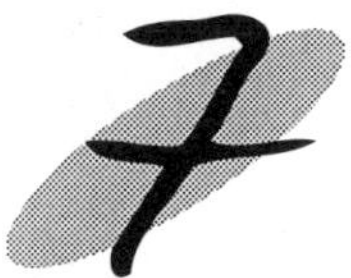

BALANCING YOUR FOOD

"I work at a fast-food place and I shovel in what I'm shoveling out. I know it isn't good for me. My skin keeps breaking out with zits because of all the grease that's flying around here."

It seems like everyone's totally confused about what's healthy or what foods promote fitness and weight loss. Just eyeball any bookstore; there are racks of books on all sorts of different diets. There's even one that says only eat pineapples—seriously! Another warns against eggs, milk and other proteins.

Who should you listen to? Medical experts, not just trendies, who can talk straight about the benefits of a balanced diet, one that includes all the food groups:

- **protein-rich** foods, such as meat, poultry, fish, dry beans, nuts and eggs;
- **dairy**, such as milk, cheese and yogurt;
- **fruit**, those sweet, crunchy or soft, sometimes peelable, portable things;
- **vegetables**—steamed, stewed or raw;
- **grains**, such as cracked wheat bread, cereal, rice, oatmeal, cornmeal and pasta—in sensible portions.

Variety is important. Don't you wonder how your dog and cat can eat the same thing every day and not lose their tiny, little minds? Not only does it prevent boredom, but a range of foods offers you the nutrition you need to get along with your life.

Doctors say adolescence is an intense anabolic time. That means you need nutrients to prevent problems later on. Besides, you're hungry, right? You need to eat.

Doctors also say that growing up requires more food, so your mom's or dad's diet may not work for you.

"I don't want to dump all over my mom, but she was a fat kid and she never wanted me to go through what she went through. But it was like she was never feeding me."

Know this: you need to eat three meals a day. No skipping. Also, slurp up calcium. The National Research Council says 11- to 24-year-olds should have 1,200 milligrams of calcium every day to prevent osteoporosis—bone shrinking. Four to five servings of any of these would set your bones straight:

- an 8-ounce glass of milk;
- 1 ounce of Swiss cheese;
- 6 ounces of plain yogurt;
- 8 ounces of frozen yogurt;
- or 4-1/2 cups of kale or collard greens.

And one more thing: There should be room in everyone's body for an occasional food fling, like milk shakes, candy bars, fried chicken or a sloppy burger. Remember, it's your total diet that counts. Junk food is OK, if you eat it in small doses and after a good meal.

"It's not so much whether you have junk food, it's whether you have only junk food that's an issue," says Dr. Ronald Barr of the Montreal Children's Hospital. If you splurge on something high in fat for lunch, ease up at dinner with a lean meat and veggies, but don't skip the meal completely, Skippy.

For more nutritional info, write for the free Food Pyramid brochure from the Consumer Information Center, Dept. 119C, Pueblo, Colorado 81009 or fax your request to 202-501-4281. Or you can download the information at http://www.pueblo.gsa.gov. Still can't decide? Call 202-501-1794.

NICOLE, 12, TALKING

"My older stepsister Sarah and I have opposite problems: she's 14 and underweight and I'm big boned, pudgy. She has to try to gain weight. A size 4 is too big for her. And when she wears her Doc Martens, she can lace them up really tight but there's still enough room around her ankles for her to put her hands into the boots.

"Sarah and another girl, Michele, who's 15, could both fit into my Levi's shorts that were tight on me. My problem is resisting sugar and candies. But I have been watching what I eat for 10 months now and I've been losing two to three pounds a month and that's a good way to lose weight.

"It was hard when I would watch Sarah eat double portions while I was cutting back. All my life it seems I always wanted more food and I was always hungry. I would beg my mom for more. But my sister would never tease me. She's a great sister. We're working as a team to get healthy.

"What I know is if you starve yourself your body will shut off and hold on to anything you eat. But if you eat three meals a day, your body will have all the nutrients you need to burn calories. As long as you don't have too much, you're OK. That's pretty easy.

"One thing that makes me want to keep eating right is that pair of shorts. I've dropped two sizes so far and I can slip them on and off without unzipping them now."

NOT SURE? THEN GET SURE

If you have a medical concern, talk to your doctor. Show him or her this book. If the doc looks confused, explain what *bodyPRIDE* means. Then doc will get it.

But you should know that this book has been reviewed by medical experts and it's based on information from Dr. Marshall Stamper of the Lindora Medical Clinics, who's worked with overweight people for 25 years. That's right, longer than you've been on this planet.

He's helped some people lose as much as 500 pounds. No kidding. One guy was so big he couldn't even get out of bed. Dr. Stamper showed him how to lose weight and keep it off by using the information in this book. The doc's an expert in the chemistry of losing weight. Like grandpa, he's cool.

SEPARATING SUGARS

There are two kinds of in-between-meals foods:

1. Healthy snacks (Angel Food cake, baked apples, fresh fruit, fruit juice, gingersnaps, lowfat chocolate milk) have vitamins and minerals, and energy in the form of calories but not too much fat or sugar. Then there are...
2. treat foods (lardy cakes, ice cream, pies, most cookies and pastries) that are high in fat and low in nutrients and should only go into your belly on special occasions, like your birthday or graduation.

If you look on the label under ingredients and the first few are sugars, such as corn syrup or fructose, and more than 30 calories per 100 come from fat, drop the package and run, do not walk, to the neighborhood frozen yogurt stand. Order a lowfat bowl dressed up with sprinkles. The small amount of added sugar in the yogurt is countered by the vitamins and minerals chillin' inside the yogurt.

Chocolate pudding is another good-for-you snack. It's a dairy product and that means it has nutrients such as calcium and protein. It's a lot better than gelatin.

Although peanut butter is a high-fat food, its fat is the better-for-your-bod unsaturated kind. You can always test a food to see if it has the good fat: unsaturated fat doesn't harden at room temperature, like your sister's hair after she over-mousses it.

EASY WAYS TO CUT IT OUT

Eating food high in fat, salt and sugar means you'll be booking an appointment with a cardiologist—a heart doc—in the future. Nutrition experts at the U.S. Department of Agriculture say that you should eat foods low in fat, saturated fat and cholesterol, and you should eat sugar, salt and sodium in moderation (yes, that means don't heap it on).

Here are other ways to get a healthy start:

- **Eat** lean meats. We're talking about the Food and Drug Administration's description that meat, poultry and seafood need to be fewer than 10 grams of fat, 4-1/2 grams or less of saturated fat and fewer than 95 milligrams of cholesterol in a typical serving (100 grams). OK with that?
- **Drink** 1% or 2% milk instead of whole milk to reduce the amount of saturated fat.
- **Use** nonstick pans and cooking sprays instead of greasing a pan with butter. A tablespoon of butter adds 102 calories and 11-1/2 grams of fat to your entree, compared to 2 calories for a spritz of cooking spray.
- **Use** vegetable oils instead of lard or bacon grease.
- **Back** off on gravy, even if it's dumped all over everything and looks so good in the school cafeteria.
- **Boil** or poach eggs. Don't fry or scramble them in oil.
- **At** fast-food places, a small hamburger has less fat than fried chicken pieces. And don't supersize your combo meal. That doubles the fat.
- **Navigate** around the fatty stuff at the salad bar: mayonnaise-heavy salads (potato salad, macaroni salad, etc.), as well as olives, cheese... you know, the heart-clogging stuff.
- **Pretzels** and air-popped popcorn are less fattening than corn or potato chips or snack crackers.
- **Bring** popcorn-flavored rice cakes into the movie theater so you can crunch along with everyone else.
- **On** the run? Bring along a small bag of raw veggies or other edibles that are low in fat. Eat these instead of fatty snacks, like peanuts, trail mix and chips.
- **Use** jam, jelly and preserves instead of butter or margarine as a bread spread.
- **Use** lowfat substitutes whenever possible. Use reduced-calorie salad dressings or make you own with low- or nonfat sour cream, mayo or yogurt blended with minced garlic, herbs or fat-free Parmesan.
- **There** are no fat-free versions of fried food—so replace them altogether with food that's baked, broiled, steamed, microwaved or roasted.
- **Eat** nonfat pinto beans that taste like beans refried in lard but without the fat. Make Thai and Indian foods with reduced-fat coconut milk.

What's your family's favorite meal? Thin it out.

- **Read** labels on packaged foods. Healthy granolas may have coconut oil—a geyser of cholesterol-raising saturated fats. "Thin" crackers may not be all they're cracked up to be. They could be shaped like vegetables, but that doesn't forgive them for being high in fat.

Want to learn how to crack the label code?

LABEL THIS

Don't let big business fool you with front-package claims of being "lite" or "reduced." Lighter than what? Reduced from what? Figure out the hidden fat. Some salad dressings have zero fat while others have 20 grams—equivalent to a slice of pizza. Some fat-free, lowfat cakes and cookies are high in calories because of added sugar. Also, your kid brother or sister may be fooled by fattening, sugar-drenched cereals or quickie dinners that lure unsuspecting young ones in with prizes and cartoonish packages.

Show big business you know better. Turn the package over and read the food label. That sounds easier than it actually is because food labels are written in code. Manufacturers make it hard to figure out exactly how much fat is hiding inside the package. It's deceptive, all right, but legal, so count on it continuing.

Let's examine your label IQ. Take a look at this one:

Nutrition Facts

Serving Size ½ cup (114g)
Servings Per Container: 4

Amount Per Serving

Calories 90	Calories from Fat 30
	% Daily Value*
Total Fat 3g	5%
Saturated Fat 0g	0%
Cholesterol 0 mg	0%
Sodium 300mg	13%
Total Carbohydrate 13g	4%
Dietary Fiber 3g	12%
Sugars 3g	
Protein 3g	

Vitamin A 80% • Vitamin C 60% • Calcium 4% • Iron 4 %

*Percent Daily Values are based on a 2,000 calorie diet. Your Daily Values may be higher or lower depending on your calorie needs:

Nutrient		2,000 Calories	2,500 Calories
Total Fat	Less than	65g	80g
Sat Fat	Less than	20g	25g
Cholesterol	Less than	300mg	300mg
Sodium	Less than	2,400mg	2,400mg
Total Carbohydrate		300g	375g
Fiber		25g	30g

Calories per gram:

What is the percentage of fat? If you think 5%, sorry but wrong! Look where it says Calories: 90. Now look where it says Calorie from Fat: 30. Each serving contains 90 calories and 30 of those calories are from fat. That means this food is 33% fat.

Yikes!

Calculator time: The federal government recommends that if we eat 2,000 calories a day, not more than 30% of those calories should come from fat. So, 2,000 calories times 30% equals 600 calories of fat per day or 67 grams of fat.

Totally confused? For more info, write for a free brochure on food labels to the Consumer Information Center, Dept. 520C, Pueblo, Colorado 81009 or fax your request to 202-501-4281. Or you can download the information at http://www.pueblo.gsa.gov. Or call 202-501-1794.

BUT BACK UP

So what's with the label stating that the "Total Fat" percentage is 5%? Goofy, we know. What that means is a single serving provides 5% of what you should eat based on your typical, 2,000-calorie diet. As if you're going to eat all your food for the day at one time.

You also have to check out the serving size. If the label says four servings per container and you gobble the whole thing, multiply everything by four.

Got it?

Great, now answer this question that we have been wondering about for years: If Mr. X takes the 11 a.m. train from New York to Washington, D.C., and Ms. Y takes the noon train from Philadelphia to Boston, why do we care what time the trains pass each other?

And while you're at it, take a look at the labels on your 10 favorite foods. Rank them in order of good-for-you (lowfat)—which go at the top of your list—to the better-watch-its, which go at the bottom.

1. ______________________ ________ (% of fat/serving)
2. ______________________ ________ (% of fat/serving)
3. ______________________ ________ (% of fat/serving)
4. ______________________ ________ (% of fat/serving)
5. ______________________ ________ (% of fat/serving)
6. ______________________ ________ (% of fat/serving)
7. ______________________ ________ (% of fat/serving)
8. ______________________ ________ (% of fat/serving)
9. ______________________ ________ (% of fat/serving)
10. ______________________ ________ (% of fat/serving)

WHO'S CHEATING?

All anyone can do is tell you that you need to eat right to feel good. The rest is up to you. Eat a fresh salad in front of your friends, then scarf a bag of candy on the way home? That's cheating. And it's not like your little brother calling up his friend and getting the codes to break through the video game levels faster. This is real cheating. You're cheating yourself.

Instead, write the U.S. Department of Agriculture for its booklets on how to buy fresh fruit (50 cents) and vegetables (again, 50 cents) at the Consumer Information Center, Dept. 319C and 320C, Pueblo, Colorado 81009. Here's the Web site address again for instant service: http://www.pueblo.gsa.gov. For more information, call 202-501-1794.

NEED A LITTLE SWEETNESS?

Here are a few recipes to satisfy you:

- **Rich chocolate pudding:**

  Whisk 2 cups lowfat milk, 2 tablespoons sugar, 2 tablespoons cornstarch and 1 tablespoon unsweetened cocoa in a saucepan until well blended. Bring to a boil over medium heat. Remove from heat. Stir in 1 square (1 oz.) chopped semisweet chocolate. Return to low heat, bring mixture to a boil, stirring constantly. Boil for 2 minutes. Stir in 1 teaspoon vanilla.

  Spoon into four 6-ounce dessert dishes. Cover with plastic wrap touching surface of pudding and refrigerate until chilled, about 3 hours. Garnish with 6 halved strawberries and reduced-fat frozen whipped topping. Try a small serving.

- **Creamy rice pudding:**

  In a 2-quart baking dish, whisk 3 cups skim milk, 1/3 cup honey, 1 teaspoon vanilla, 1/4 teaspoon ground nutmeg and 1/4 teaspoon ground cinnamon. Stir in 1-1/2 cup cooked rice. Microwave on high for 10 minutes. Stir well, then microwave on high for another 10 minutes. Whisk in 1/2 cup fat-free egg substitute. Microwave on high for 2 minutes. Stir and let stand for at least 10 minutes to thicken. Serve warm or cold. Garnish with peach slices.

BESIDES GREAT TASTE

For the most part, being fit means staying away from those gooey, sugary treats that get trapped in your teeth and cause cavities. Steer clear of them and you'll be looking at less time in the dentist's chair. That means no more Novocaine shots, dental drilling and drooling in public because your mouth's numb afterward.

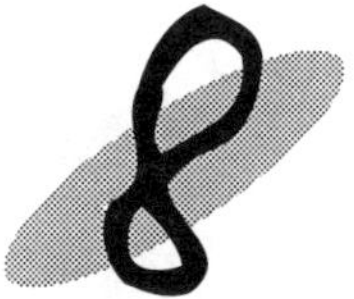

ALL THOSE WORKING PARTS

You're one great machine. The bones, the blood, the muscle, the organs, the this, the that. There's nothing quite like you.

OK, stop admiring yourself (at least for a moment or two; we know it's hard). Besides realizing how wonderful your body is, you also know that you have to keep it fueled. The speediest Porsche needs fuel and so do you.

Food is your fuel. It provides nutrients. But it doesn't always give your body everything it needs. So to help it out, pump in some high-quality multiple vitamins with mineral supplements. They help your body absorb the good stuff in your food and prevent you from getting nutritional deficiencies, like scurvy or other diseases that may even make your teeth decay and fall out.

ABCs OF VITAMINS

From health class, you found out that A, C and D are vitamins and iron, sodium and magnesium are minerals. You also learned that:

- **Vitamins** are compounds that help the body use proteins, carbohydrates, fats and minerals.
- **They're** important for the formation of red blood cells and other body functions. They make you more mentally alert and fight infection.
- **Minerals** are elements that help your body's processes, including blood clotting, muscle movement and fluid balance. When it comes to bones, the mineral calcium plays an important structural role.

OK, so how do you get all these must-haves into your body? It's easy. There are multivitamins available that pack most of what you need into one pill or capsule that you can swallow every morning to jump-start your day.

You're set. Now you can go back to admiring yourself.

VITAMIN TRICKS

Pete says, "It's hard to remember to take vitamins. Like, they're so small, who even sees them? It seems like I remember them on the way to school, and I hit myself on the forehead and say, `Doh!', just like Homer Simpson. Now I leave the vitamins in the drawer where the knives and forks are, so when I reach in there in the morning, I see them. You gotta make it obvious."

Want some other tips?

If you don't like the aftertaste of a vitamin, take it in between your meal so the last, lingering taste you have is your food.

If you put your vitamins in the freezer for at least a few hours before you take them, your body will absorb them more slowly and the taste won't be as strong.

Figure out if you're a capsule or a pill person. Then down that type.

POP QUIZ

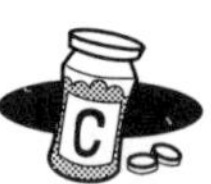

Did you take your vitamin today? Smart. Now check it off here, on your vitamin entry You'll see this again on your Daily Action Plan. Your what? We'll get to it. No hurry.

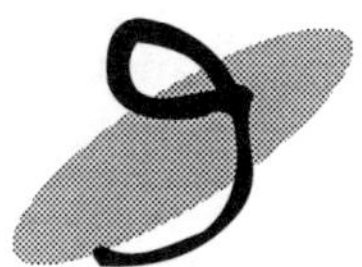

SEEING IT HAPPEN

Your Daily Action Plan is your buddy. It's warm, cuddly and loves to go for rides in the family car...

All right, it may not be all that, but it can help you. It's your best friend when it comes to reaching your goals. It won't do the work for you but it's a good tool. Your DAP (Daily Action Plan=DAP) helps you stay informed about the days that add up to become your week, month, year, life. By writing down what you do on your DAP every day, you'll have a record of what you did and where you're heading. If something punches a hole in your plan, record it here. Instead of getting zapped again, you'll know what to do and what not to do.

So what does this DAP look like? An example of a DAP is on page 53.

1. Enter today's day and date—like, *Duh!*
2. Write down everything you ate, whether you're trying to lose weight or not. This helps you keep track of those all-important three meals a day. Do this right after you've eaten, while the food is fresh in your belly and the info is fresh in your head. That way, you won't have to go fumbling through your brain to remember what you inhaled nine hours before.

- **BREAKFAST** ....

  ....

  Healthy snack ....

  ....
- **LUNCH** ....

  ....

  Healthy snack ....

  ....
- **DINNER** ....

  ....

  Occasional Dessert ....

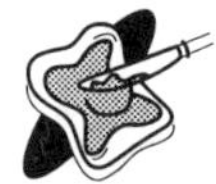

3. Scribble down the number of carbohydrates and fats you've eaten. Carbs are starchy stuff like bread and rice. And you know what fats are.

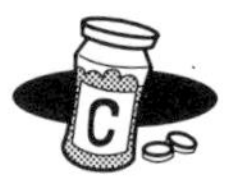

4. Check this box to say, "Yep, I've chomped my necessary vitamins today."

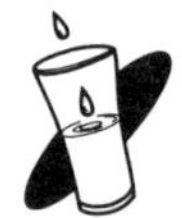

5. Water report goes here. Also record other liquids you've downed beyond the required Big 64 oz. of H_20.

6. Weigh yourself every morning after going to the bathroom but before you put on your clothes. Yes, you're naked (or at least close); we told you this would be fun. Enter the proud number here.

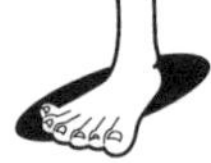

7. Chalk in here the zillions (OK, thousands) of steps you took per your step counter.

8. Now, it's big boast time. Write down all the exercise you did during the whole day—what it was, how long you did it, how sweaty you got (this last one's optional).

9. Imagine one of those positive "I am great" statements appearing on your brain's computer screen. Then write it down here. Try for a different message every day.

10. Your dream is publicized here.

11. The steps you'll take today to reach your dream are outlined here.

12. Anticipate any challenges you will face today that may dent your dream. What could get in the way? What's your plan to get past it? Remember: Don't let any person or any excuse torpedo your plan.

13. Reward time: Write here what reward you'll give yourself for being so awesome.

Tip: Fill out your DAP every day to chart your success. Look at past ones to see how far you've come toward your dream. If you've made progress, keep it up. And fix any problems. The excellent thing about keeping a DAP is that you'll know what works and what doesn't work for you.

DAILY ACTION PLAN

• Day ❶ ....

• Date ❶ ....

• BREAKFAST ❷ ....

....

Healthy snack ....

....

• LUNCH ❷ ....

....

Healthy snack ....

....

• DINNER ❷ ....

....

Occasional Dessert ....

How Many Carbs? ❸

How Much Fat? ❸

Vitamins?

❹ ☐ Yep! ☐ Nope.

How much Water? ❺

Weight? ❻

How Many Steps? ❼

• For Exercise, I ❽ ....

....

• I Am Great because ❾ ....

....

• My Dream is ❿ ....

....

• To reach it, today I will ⓫ ....

....

• If ⓬ .... happens, I will ....

....

• My reward today is ⓭ ....

O.K. So Instead I'm On www.bodypride.com

GUARANTEED...OR YOUR ANGER BACK

You'll feel better every day if you:

- **dump** some soap and water on your face and body and clean up those greasy spots.
- **tell** yourself how lovable (and loving) you are.
- **wear** clothes that fit comfortably.
- **eat** three balanced meals.
- **learn** at least one new thing (knowing that number 4 follows number 3 doesn't, uh, count).
- **don't** owe anyone any money.
- **drink** 64 ounces of water to minimize any cola pollutants and make your eyes brighter.
- **wave** at your parents. Smiles are good. Hugs are better.
- **help** another teen by listening or giving good advice based on your experience.
- **be** aware of what's happening elsewhere in the world. Newspaper? News broadcast? City council meeting? Plug in somewhere.
- **scramble** around and burn off energy.
- **reward** yourself for building positive habits that will benefit you for life.
- ______________________________

  ____

  ____

(Add to your list)

ODAY, 14, TALKING

"My name is Oday. It's an Arabic name that means someone with strong willpower. No one can peer-pressure me or tell me what to do unless I want to do it. If I'm going to do something, I'll do it right and I don't stop after only a week.

"I had low self-esteem until the 6th grade when I stopped letting people walk all over me and make fun of me. If an adult has low self-esteem, it's much harder for them to raise it because they have had it for a long time. But teens can do it.

"If I'm feeling down, I talk to people who give me a hug and who don't say I'm bad just because I didn't do everything exactly right. And I say to myself, 'You're going to do it' and I tell myself how good I'll feel when I've done something good for me.

"If I'm trying to make a change, I make a Daily Action Plan. In the beginning, you can't go from doing something wrong your whole life to immediately doing it right. It's steps. It's something I can do on my own.

"It's like working out. I've never been into sports but I didn't want to be weak so I started slow and built up. Wrestling, running, bicycling and the stepper get me in shape.

"If you do a plan right—because you want to do it—it can make a humongous change."

Part 2

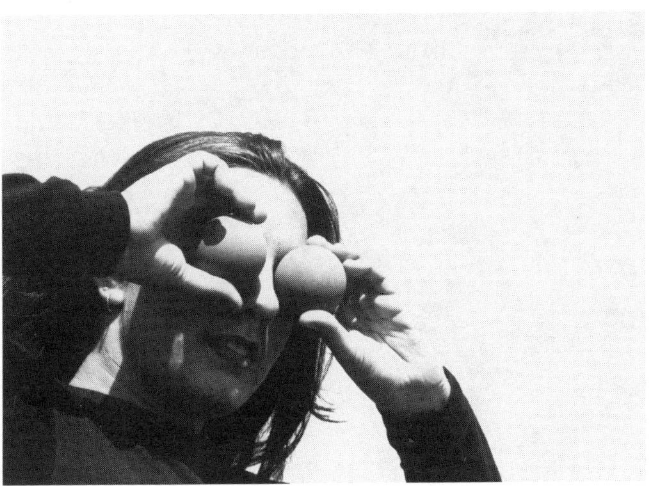

MESSING UP

In this section, you'll learn how to recover after you've slipped from your plan, how to deal with pressures from friends or families, and why bouncing back and forgiving yourself is part of being a successful human.

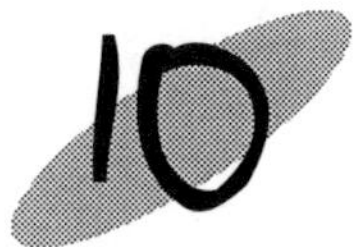

TAKING A DIVE

Mark Lenzi won a gold medal for diving in the 1992 Olympics in Barcelona. Wow.

Then he blew it. He went overboard on booze and junk food. "I was a tub," he said.

He dove into savings and after a few years, came up dry. Needing cash, he even considered pawning his gold medal. Not Wow.

Mark admits now—after successfully pulling himself back into form and winning a bronze medal in the springboard competition in the 1996 Olympics in Atlanta—that his slide was because he wasn't prepared for the future. Mark just thought that if he won in Barcelona, he was set for life.

The way he figured it, advertisers would pay him big bucks to smile on their cereal boxes. TV producers would bring him juicy offers. Fans would buy tickets just to hear him talk.

Sure, Mark thought, he could float on this Olympic cloud forever. Right. After a few months, he came down with a fat thud. Then he disappeared from view altogether.

"You start believing you're God's gift to the world," Mark said. "The next day, no one knows you."

Mark never stopped to consider what he would do after '92. A lot of athletes and other successful people feel this letdown after a big win. They have reached their dream and, they ask, "Now what?"

DREAM AGAIN

They need to say to themselves, "All Right! Congrats, you did it. You made it happen." Then they need to ask, "What is my new dream?"

Mark started scrambling for something: He wanted to be a pilot, but that didn't fly. His coach said Mark would change his mind all the time. "He was a mess," is the way the coach put it.

What did Mark need?

It took three years, but Mark rediscovered he was still great at diving; and if he focused on that again, he could have another shot at the Olympics. Everyone called him the "comeback kid," but few actually believed he'd win a spot on the '96 U.S. team. Think about it—all the other athletes had spent the last three years training. They hadn't gained 30 pounds or stayed clear of the water like Mark.

Determined, he headed off to the Olympic trails in Indianapolis with this message in his head: "You're the best diver in the world." And he came through. Mark did a flawless reverse 3-1/2 somersault tuck and won one of two springboard spots on the team.

He kept the momentum going at the Olympics in Atlanta. He came from behind to grab that bronze, even though many people had written him off.

With that new medal in hand, a polished reputation and, especially, the knowledge that he could come back, Mark returned to his home in Indiana sure that he wouldn't belly flop again.

"This time," he said, "I have a plan."

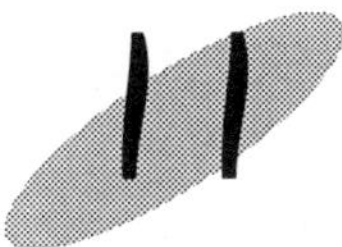

SETBACKS

You go to the movies with your friends. They buy Snickers and a tub of popcorn. You don't want to make a big announcement that you're watching what you scarf so you order one of those monster sodas and a side of popcorn. Before you know it, this lousy feeling sticks to you like gum to a theater seat.

You think you've blown it and you'll never get fit.

Relax. You just drank a soda and ate some popcorn. Your friends aren't going to ditch you. The world is not crashing to an end. The rain forest is not being devastated....actually, it is (a really bad thing), but that's a different story.

But blowing a diet for a day, missing an appointment, forgetting to study are all part of living. You will never be perfect—sorry, but it's true—and no one should expect you to be. Perfection won't get you to your goal, being smart will. And being smart means understanding that one mistake, one setback doesn't push you all the way back to the very beginning.

You can pick up where you fell off. It's no big deal. Pretend there's a giant blackboard and you have a huge eraser. Rub out the mistake, misstep or misunderstanding. Then get on with your plan. Slapping yourself around over small things will take all the fun out of achieving the big things.

If you notice that you're using that eraser a lot, see if you can find a pattern: a specific place, event or person that seems to dust your dream. Being aware of the temptation means you won't fall for it again.

Oh, and when you have a sec, write your congressman about the rain forest. Pollution, too.

"Learn from your mistakes so you don't repeat them, that's what I try to do. I know I have the power not to keep going around and around on the same old, broken down ride."

REBOUNDS

Jamal will tell you he really fouled up his fitness plan:

"I got my step counter Thursday night and started counting my steps. The next day, I logged 9,567 steps. Saturday, I left my pedometer at home when I went to Lollapalooza. I stayed 11 hours and I didn't drink very much water. I know that if I'd brought my pedometer, I would have added 10,000 steps. I'm re-motivated and have begun my fitness program again, right this time, by drinking more water and using my pedometer."

How do you think Jamal will do?

His chances will be greater if he figures out what traps may be lying in wait for him and then works out a strategy to avoid them. Like, before he heads off to the next concert, he can think, "Tickets, cash, pedometer...check" and he can chug water until he has to leave home. That way, he's set for the day.

TAKE A CHANCE

How would you react to these situations:

1. Your friends are heading out for a fast-food pigout. What are you going to do?

   Your answer:____

   ____

   Here's another: Be part of the group, make a good choice from the menu (like grilled chicken with the mayo or secret sauce scraped off), don't breathe in when that great French fries smell comes your way, and remind yourself that healthy eating is about making the right choices every time you eat.

2. Your friends are plowing through McTub o' Lard while you're checking to see how many fat grams are in the McHealthy Delux. You're starting to feel like an outsider. How come they can eat anything they want and you can't? You're feeling left out and deprived. What do you do?

   Your answer:____

   ____

Another answer: Remember that this is temporary. When the meal's been wolfed down and empty wrappers litter the table, no one will remember who ate what. Except you'll be feeling rather superior that you didn't bend. Your plan to be healthy wasn't fezzed, frazzed, dregged, bluzzed or blasted over something as fleeting as fast food.

3. Another sticky spot is the school cafeteria and we don't mean the goo on the floor. The stuff in those big steel trays may have lots of fats—unfortunately many foods everywhere do. The cheapest thing is the Xtra Cheeze Macaroni and you're always short on coins. What do you eat?

   Your answer:____

   ____

   Another answer: If this happens a lot, bring food from home. That way, you can control what you're eating—good, nutritious stuff wrapped up and looking appetizing.

Whatever your plan is, you'll be doing things differently and it may not seem comfortable all the time, but if you know in the long run that it's positive, stick with it. It's kind of like flossing. When you were smaller and had big gaps between your teeth, it didn't seem to make sense to saw string between those gaps. But you knew that if you got in the habit of brushing and flossing, you wouldn't have a toothless smile when you're ancient, say 40. Good habits pay off over and over again.

BLANKING OUT

Sometimes, instead of thinking through a situation and making a good choice, you may go temporarily unconscious. The result? Your old habits will creep back in.

You know what we're talking about: you sit down in front of the TV to watch a few minutes of basketball and suddenly, it's lights out and your math book is right where you left it: next to your notebook paper that's as blank as the look in your eyes after a marathon of tube-gazing.

What happened? Was your brain kidnapped? (Any ransom notes scattered around the room?)

You slipped into automatic pilot and flew in the wrong direction.

And you're wondering, "How come I can be so disciplined sometimes, then other times, I'm zzzzzzzing with my mouth open, drooling like a Great Dane?"

Here's the deal: All actions have consequences...you know A equals B. This becomes That. Boy Meets Girl (heh-heh, sorry). Think about what you're doing now and how that's going to affect you in a few minutes...hours....or days. Would you really trade off your health and good looks tomorrow for a doughnut today?

OTHER PEOPLE

You're surrounded by people who are making decisions that are good for them. That doesn't mean their plans are always right for you. Sometimes, without thinking about it, friends and family sabotage your plans. Your friends urge you to go shopping instead of studying. Your sister offers to drive you and your pals to the movies when you should be working. Your dad yells, "it's Pizza-time!" just as you're heading to the gym.

"My mom is obsessed with her weight. When she gets tempted for something fattening like a chili cheese dog she orders one for me when I'm not even hungry and asks me to save her a bite. It's like asking me to smoke so she can inhale the second-hand smoke. It's not healthy for me."

What can you do about it?

Keeping quiet and feeling crummy about it is the wrong turn, way wrong. Open, honest talk is always the best direction. Find a good place to talk to [fill in his/her name] and:

- **State** the problem. Maybe say something like, "I really want to [say your dream] but it's not easy. I need your help."
- **Explain** how you feel about the way they're acting. "I'm wrenched because I know you care about me, but some of the things you've been doing make it tough for me to reach my goal."
- **Detail** what you want and don't assume everyone knows it. "Instead of doing something that goes against what I want to do, let's do something together."
- **Lay out** what you're hoping for and what steps you're taking to get there. "I'm going to do this right and I want to know you're really with me on it."

OTHER PEOPLE'S PROBLEMS

There may be people out there—maybe even "friends"—who like it when you don't feel good about yourself because it makes them feel better about themselves. Don't live your life for them. You'll spot selfish people this way: If they try to stop you from making a change that's good for you, it's because they don't want what's best for you. Think hard about what kind of friends they really are...and be true to yourself first.

"My friend Brianna gets straight As. When I told her that I'm getting a tutor to get help, she told me she thought that was dumb. Why should she care if it will help me?"

When you feel good about yourself, some of your friends may resent you. They may think you're stuck up or trying to leave them in the dust and move on to other friends. Let them know that you're loyal to them as long as they support you. Tell them, too, that you'll help them with stuff they're working on.

"I see my friends doing stuff that's just not for me. It's not like I want everything they have."

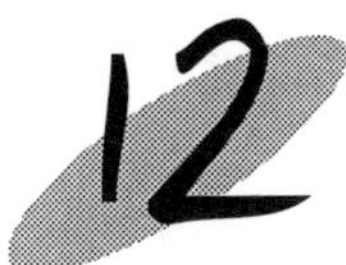

EXCUSES, EXCUSES

Have you ever lied to yourself? You know, told yourself that a problem really isn't there or made up excuses why you did something rather than facing the truth? These are tricks to avoid bad feelings, hard situations or painful truths. After all, as long as we don't see a problem, we don't have to fix it.

Have you ever said something like: "It wasn't my fault. My friends made me do it" or "I had no choice"? Sounds pretty convincing, right? Well, maybe. But they're still not true. And every time you use an excuse, you push yourself backward into babyland.

THEY'RE EVERYWHERE

Excuses pop up for every occasion, like:

Relationships:

- "He isn't nice to me but I know he loves me."
- "What I don't know won't hurt me."

Families:

- "Things could be different if my family weren't so uptight."
- "I deserve this. Everyone else gets to have fun. It's my turn."

Health:

- "I'm not gaining weight, the dryer shrunk them."
- "It's not really junk food. Even some athletes eat this stuff."

School:

- "I could have aced that test but I didn't have time to study."
- "I'll make it up tomorrow."

Change:

- "I would like to change that about myself, but I'm too busy and stressed to try anything new right now."
- "It's OK if I don't do it this one time. It's Friday/Saturday/Sunday night. It's my birthday. It's a holiday."

All-occasion:

- ◆ "It's no big deal."
- ◆ "Yes, but [fill in the rest]."

All of these excuses take your power away from you. You blame your parents, friends, brother, sister, teacher, coach...everyone but the person who's really in charge: You.

By being straight with yourself—and not allowing flimsy excuses or denial to fog your vision—you can change the way you live.

Fight excuses and denial with these five weapons:

1. Go ahead and admit that excuses are following you. When they pop up, stop yourself mid-sentence and say, "Wait. I'm in charge. How do I want this to work out?"
2. Douse negative thoughts with positive ones. If you're thinking, "Skipping a class is not going to kill me," change that thought to a question, such as, "Are the few minutes of fun I'll get from doing something else really worth the bad way I'll feel tomorrow when the consequences come my way?" This reminds you that there's a price to pay.
3. Avoid repeating the same defeating self-talk by understanding the problems these little lies have created for you in the past. Look for bad patterns and sidestep them.
4. Be aware of the "Not Me" syndrome. If you find yourself thinking that some of this doesn't apply to you and so you can ignore it, look closely: denial may be covering up the truth. You want to have the courage to examine your motives, understand your reactions and learn life's lessons along the way.
5. Giving excuses and denying a problem doesn't stop overnight. It's an ongoing process. There will be times when they get the best of you. That's OK. Admit that you slipped, learn from the experience and accept that you made a bad choice. Then try not to repeat it.

"All excuses are worthless. Don't try it; do it! If I blow it, I don't even say why. I just admit it. 'Mom, I'm sorry I forgot to pick up Benny from daycare. I messed up and won't do it again' is a lot stronger than whining about the flat tire on my friend's car."

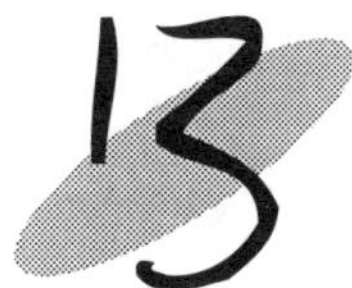

HARD TO IGNORE

If the thought of attacking the neighbor's yard, teepeeing someone's car or wrecking a wall with graffiti jumps into your head, then think about this: You don't have to do any of that stuff. Stop before you act. Think it through, weigh the fallout—"Hello, Mrs. Mitchell, we have bad news. Your son Dennis is down here at the police station"—and figure out something better to do with your time.

Sometimes, it's not even your bad idea. Friends may prod you into doing something you shouldn't with, "Oh, come on. It'll be a blast and who'll know?"

There are some places that tug on you to lose all control—"I always overspend at the music store" or "I always get carried away at the all-you-can-eat places."

The power of your life shouldn't be in the hands of your friends or anything else. You have ultimate control—especially over your body. The main thing to remember is that cravings and impulses are suggestions, not commands. You don't have to give in. If they're bad for you, zap 'em.

TAKE A CHANCE

Which people, places and events seem to make you blow off your goal? Example: "When I'm busy, I want fast food so I don't have to prepare a healthy meal." Or "When I'm tired, I get edgy, lose my temper and start a fight."

Make a list of ways you get off track, then find a way to get back on.

When I'm....	I crave....	When what I could do is....
___________	___________	___________
___________	___________	___________
___________	___________	___________
___________	___________	___________
___________	___________	___________

TRICKS FOR STAYING IN CONTROL

Before you do anything that might harm your progress, STOP!

Stall. Visualize a stop sign.

Take a deep breath. This will give you a chance to think things through.

Observe your behavior. What are you thinking of doing? Why? What would it accomplish? How are you feeling? Are you hungry, tired, angry, lonely? What's really going on? Is this a habit that's not good for you?

Plan your action. Shift the focus away from That Thing That's Bad For You by doing something positive: take a walk, call a friend, listen to music, head to the gym, go dancing, work on a project. You'll find that if you wait it out your temptation will pass. This is the rare occasion when stall tactics can work in your favor.

Whatever you do, don't sit around and think and think and think about how powerful your cravings are. That's called obsessing, and it's a big waste of time.

Instead, calmly consider what will happen if you cave in. Ask yourself how you'll feel tomorrow if you give into your impulses today. Do you really want to sleep in and miss your job interview? What about the car or tuition you were saving for? It's a good idea to review your motivation index cards (from page 11) to remind yourself what your goals are, that you can make it happen.

"I ask myself, 'What is it I really want?' Will doing this make me feel better?"

HAVE A PROBLEM WITH IMPULSE BUYING?

- **Before** you head out, remember your goal. Make a list of what you really need and don't waver no matter how great something seems.
- **Never** shop when you're hungry, stressed or tired. You'd be an easy target to some fast-talking salesperson ("It's perfect for you!"), an enticing package or something fattening from the food court.
- **Steer** clear of danger zones, those spots that always lure you into buying something that's not necessary.
- **Shop** with friends with willpower who will help you avoid temptation (ask them ahead of time to help you stay strong). And be a stand-up person and do the same for them.
- **Shop** less and buy more. The more often you visit the store, the more likely you'll buy junk you don't need.

HOW ABOUT IMPULSE EATING?

- **Choose** restaurants carefully. If you're not sure they serve healthy food, call ahead. Avoid all-you-can eat or big food places that encourage over-stuffing. Don't look at the menu—it will just offer you choices that you don't want to make. Instead, tell the server what you'd like.

  Speak up and be specific—say you want your entree the way you like it, broiled, baked or grilled, with steamed veggies and a salad with lowfat dressing on the side. Or whatever. Also, tell the server in advance to ditch the dessert tray. Don't be shy about it. Inexpensive chains and fancy-smancy places all want to please health-conscious customers.
- **Let** friends and family know you're speeding down the health track. Instead of socializing at a restaurant or fast-food joint, suggest a place outside, away from the scents of a greasy grill.
- **Be** creative. Even the Lard Family drops something on the table that doesn't clog your arteries. Examine all the offerings and figure out how to avoid the unhealthy minefields. Don't let anyone else's appetite affect your health. And yeah, you can do it with diplomacy. No need to offend your host or your family with sneers and lines like, "You eat this crap?"
- **Build** time into your day for breakfast, even if it means getting up 10 minutes earlier. Unload some cereal pieces in a bowl, drown 'em in milk and sit down long enough to enjoy it. On the way out the door, grab a piece of fruit or a container of yogurt. Your easy-to-make meal is much cheaper and better for you than the street vendor stuff your neighbor Louie gobbles on the way to work.
- **Get** rid of anything that downs your plan: marshmallows under the mattress; ice cream sandwiches stuffed behind the Tupperware of mystery meat in the freezer; jumbo bags of Halloween candy bought "early" in April. You get the idea.
- **Bring** your lunch to school or work. And avoid vending machines and snack lines, unless they're stocked with fruit and juice.
- **At** parties, always avoid alcohol (it's illegal if you're not 21, remember). Not only does booze contain worthless calories, but it lowers your metabolism, clouds your judgment and softens your resistance. Stick to diet sodas or mineral water. Live a little: add a lime wedge.
- **Steer** clear of buffets, party platters, tubs of chips or trays of cookies. They're easier to resist if you find someone irresistible to talk to. Eat before you arrive so you won't be lightheaded and say something like, "Nice ears."

WHATEVER...

Whatever obstacles you face, remember you always have a choice as to how to react. You can choose to feel bad and beat yourself up or you can use the experience as an opportunity to learn and grow. Your attitude can change a spiraling loss into a high-flying glory.

TIRED? CONFUSED?

Does it seem like you slip up more at the end of the day when you're beat? Are your defenses down when you're stressed, angry or on deadline? Do you tend to lose motivation or focus on the weekends, holidays, summer vacation? Can your friends push you off track?

Recognizing patterns will help you become more aware of your soft spots. Is there a way to pace yourself or build exercise into your day so that you don't feel so vulnerable or rundown at dinner time? Can you come up with other ways of reacting to stress or anger? Could you structure your non-school days so they're no longer a time for blowing it? Can you talk to a friend about supporting your efforts?

"Adults always say that kids have no discipline but we stick to things as much as they do, it's just that we're not doing the same stuff they're doing."

THESE THREE

People who make it have three common traits:

1. They believe it's possible to improve their situation. What you do influences the results you get.
2. They really want to improve. Not everybody wants to make their life better. Sometimes we become so comfortable that it's hard to change. Do you really want to change something? Are there any hidden payoffs to keeping everything as it is? Your friends may like you a certain way and they may threaten to ditch you if you change. But what's best for you?
3. Achievers are also persistent in improving their situation. If what you're doing is right for you, refuse to give up.

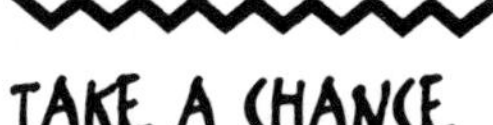

TAKE A CHANCE

Write down three accomplishments that you're really proud of:

1. ______________________________
2. ______________________________
3. ______________________________

List three specific skills, abilities, attitudes or behaviors that contributed to each of those successes:

1. a)__________ b)__________ c)__________
2. a)__________ b)__________ c)__________
3. a)__________ b)__________ c)__________

For example: education, experience, exercise, stick-to-it-tive-ness, determination, typing skills, talking skills, boldness, enthusiasm, give-it-a-try attitude, talent, and on and on and on.

Review your new list. See? You've got what it takes.

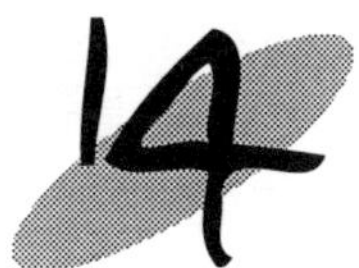

SLOW-MOTION SUICIDE

A few months before his 18th birthday, James Patterson borrowed his dad's Suburban, took a 12-pack of beer from the fridge, gathered up seven of his best friends and headed out to the desert for an overnight campout.

On the way home the next day, the Chevy flipped over. James' friends, along with all the empty beer cans, spilled onto the highway. Three friends were seriously injured. Four teenage boys died. When James was able to get out of the car, all he could do was stare at the bodies.

"It's my fault," the high school senior said later. "I've killed my friends." James' blood alcohol level was more than twice the legal limit for adults. One of the survivors said, "If James was drunk, we were all drunk, because we didn't realize that James was too drunk to drive."

James pleaded guilty to four counts of vehicular manslaughter and two counts of felony drunk driving. His sentence was light because of his age. He spent 120 days in jail, beginning the day after his final exams, and 120 days in alcohol rehab. During an emotional court session, he faced the parents of those who died. They told James how his actions changed their lives, that their pain and loss would be with them forever.

Today James wears a tattoo with the initials PJTJ, to forever remember his four friends who died in the desert: "Pig" (who was nicknamed after Piggy in "Lord of the Flies"), Jono, Tony and John.

THE STRAIGHT FACTS

Even low doses of alcohol screw with your judgment. The National Council on Alcoholism and Drug Dependence (NCA) says a third of teens in long-term juvenile institutions were under the influence of alcohol when they were arrested. Half of teen victims said they were drunk or stoned when a crime was committed against them. And it's believed that alcohol is involved in two-thirds of sexual assaults and date rapes.

Is this what fun is?

Alcohol changes your personality and ability to learn and remember information. Students with Ds or Fs drink three times as much as those who earn As, says the NCA.

Teens who binge drink—down five or more drinks in a row—say they're usually alone when they drink, and do it when they're upset or bored.

Is this what fun is?

Alcohol's bottom line: It damages your insides (like your brain and liver, the important parts). It can cause respiratory problems, depression and death. Booze makes you dependent. Oh, and if you're pregnant and drinking, plan on delivering a baby with fetal-alcohol syndrome.

Mothers Against Drunk Driving say drunks kill more than 2,000 American teens every year. Alcohol-related accidents are the leading cause of death for 15- to 24-year olds. About half of teen drownings, fires, suicides and homicides are related to drinking.

Is this what fun is?

Call the National Council on Alcoholism and Drug Dependence at 800-NCA-CALL or 202-737-8122 for information on how to prevent alcohol-related tragedies. If someone you know needs help because of a drinking problem, call the Alanon Alateen number listed in the phone book for information and nearby classes.

SNUFF IT OUT

If you wait until you're in your 20s before you drink alcohol, take drugs or use tobacco, you're more likely to be a responsible drinker, more likely to stay away from drugs and tobacco, and less likely to ever have a problem. What's the rush? Don't you have enough going on?

BUTT OUT

Now this is going to make you angry. The most popular brands of cigarettes among adults are the generic brands, you know, the cheap stuff in the plain wrapping that isn't advertised. The most popular brands of cigarettes among teens are Marlboro, Camel and Newport—the three brands that spend billions each year on advertising. You're too smart to fall for their line.

But this is the maddening part. The tobacco industry knows that 90% of adults who smoke started when they were in their teens and that it's highly unlikely that a person who reaches 21 without smoking will ever start. So they panic and do everything they can to get teens to light up. And they've worked the angles pretty well. About 3,000 teens start smoking every day. The numbers have been going up since 1992, reversing a 16-year decline.

Here's the craziest part. The tobacco industry slipped up and let one of its reports get out into the public. It says they target "teens who aren't leaders, who don't feel optimistic about the future," when they design promotions. They give "loser teens" free packs of cigarettes to get them hooked on nicotine, not to mention the other 4,000 harmful substances cigs carry.

And these teens are falling for it. They keep letting these fat cats make big bucks off them. The tobacco industry already rakes in $50 billion—as in BILLION—a year. Isn't that enough? Stop with the handouts. Hey, if you want to give your money away, how about making a donation to your favorite charity? It's way healthier.

Remember the 3,000 teens who start smoking every year? One thousand of them will die because of smoking-related diseases. The Federal Drug Administration says more Americans die from tobacco than die from AIDS, car accidents, murders, suicides, alcohol and drugs combined.

Seven out of 10 teens regret that they smoke. "Smoking is the most important public health problem facing us and the most preventable," says the Federal Drug Administration commissioner.

No butts about it.

"My boyfriend is a football player and I love him, but there are a few things that I turn my back to. Although I'd like to think he's perfect, he's not. He smokes, which I don't like. He never does it around me, but for any other boy he would get a minus one on my chart for that."

FIND THE SOURCE

The American Lung Association has a 20-day program that will help you quit smoking. Find the number in the phone book or dial 800-586-4872 for info.

Why do you smoke? The National Cancer Institute answers that question in its free (we like free) brochure, available by writing to the Consumer Information Center, Dept. 533C, Pueblo, Colorado 81009 or fax your request to 202-501-4281. Or you can download the information instantly (we like instantly) at http://www.pueblo.gsa.gov. Or call 202-501-1794.

And, the Federal Drug Administration has information on gum, patches and other ways to help smokers quit. Write to or message the same address above.

INSTANT BAD NEWS ABOUT STUFF THAT SMOKES

- **Tobacco**: It stains your teeth, fingers, clothes. It burns your hair, furniture, clothes. It gives you bad breath. It makes you winded and your hair stink. Does that make you attractive?

  It's expensive and it's illegal to sell cigarettes to minors in all 50 states.

  And forget that truthless message sent out by those "slim" cigarettes: smoking doesn't wipe out your appetite or help you lose weight. Actually, smoking teens are more likely to be overweight than non-smoking teens. Tobacco in your mouth doesn't mean you won't eat chocolate. Besides, it smokes up your insides and pollutes the air around you—like we need more of that.

- **Cannabis**—marijuana, pot, dope, grass, weed: Studies show it can reduce your concentration and motivation and increase your appetite. It damages your lungs and pulmonary system.

STEROIDS

Canadian sprinter Ben Johnson had his 1988 Summer Olympic gold medal for the 100-meter dash stripped away after tests showed he was on steroids. He—and others—took steroids to increase muscle and reduce fat. It cost him.

Steroid abusers may make the team but they forfeit their long-term dreams. The synthetic version of the hormone testosterone plays havoc with your liver and kidneys

Ever experience sharp groin pain? You can expect a lot of that with steroids. Steroids pummel your heart and other vital organs, and stunt bone growth. Boys can get enlarged prostate glands. Girls develop male characteristics.

Did we mention steroids are illegal, sold on the black market and made in motel rooms and warehouses without any concern for potency or purity?

The Federal Drug Administration puts steroids in the same habit-forming category as cocaine, heroin and LSD. Courts are giving stiff sentences for dealing. Athletes are vigorously speaking out against it. Muscle & Fitness magazine has written about the dangers. The Olympic game organizers, National Football League and National Collegiate Athletic Association closely monitor and discipline for its use.

It's funny that steroids are called "performance enhancers" and a "health formula," considering the end results: Abusers go into comas and die. And there's also the problem with 'roid rage, where your anger veers out of control, which is bad news in any book.

Why accept the unhealthy consequences, as well as the disgrace of being eliminated from competition or arrested for using steroids? Instead, be smart, sports-wise. The key to bigger muscles is exercise. When you exercise, proteins get into your muscles and make them bigger. Stop working out and they shrink.

The American Dietetic Association also reminds us that:

- **To** prevent feeling weak or tired, eat iron-packed lean red meats, fish and poultry, green leafy vegetables, fortified cereals and dried beans (legumes). Vitamin C (from oranges, strawberries, cantaloupe, tomato, broccoli, cabbage, cauliflower and green peppers) are iron-stackers as well. Iron carries oxygen to your blood.
- **Eating** cookies, candy or other sweet things will not give you a boost before an athletic event.
- **When** you absolutely, positively must have something sweet, vanilla wafers, gingersnaps, graham crackers and fruit bars are best. Carry these snacks with you so you don't go mental after a workout and eat the runt kid next to you.
- **Athletes** only need slightly more nutrients and calories than nonathletes. So don't let a coach tell you to eat tons of unnecessary stuff.

- **Drink** water before, during and after you work out and sweat. Limiting liquids to make weight dulls your performance, cuts your concentration and hurts your kidneys.
- **Calcium** (milk, yogurt, cheese) makes bones strong and helps them grow. Your bones absorb most of their calcium in your teen years and early 20s. Don't skimp and you'll grow to your maximum height, Shaq.
- **High-fat** foods (mayonnaise, peanut butter, fried foods, cheesy pizza, bacony hamburgers, you guess the rest) make you slug-like because they take a long time for your body to digest. Avoid these—especially before a big athletic performance.

The publication, "Steroids and Sports," is available free from the Consumer Information Center, Pueblo, Colorado 81009 or fax your request to 202-501-4281. Or you can download the information at http://www.pueblo.gsa.gov. Call 202-501-1794.

DRUGS

You're no baby. You've already made a personal decision about drugs. You're smart enough to figure out the fallout. You're strong enough not to fall for that peer pressure excuse. You've got your eye on the future.

But maybe a friend of yours is struggling with the idea of drugs. Tell him or her that drugs are risky. One bad experience can change your life, ruin your chance to get a job or go to college. Drugs affect all your systems—circulatory, respiratory, nervous, reproductive. There's nausea, fatigue, brain damage, comas, convulsions, death.

Harsh truth: People with low self-esteem fall for drugs. Don't hang out with them. Saying, "Everyone's doing it" is second-grade stuff.

"Every day in every class, there is always someone high. Guaranteed. Some are quiet and keep to themselves. Others act loud. Sometimes they disrupt class by talking out of turn, getting out of their seats at inappropriate times or giving irrelevant answers to questions. Students sometimes clue the teacher in by saying, 'He's f-a-d-e-d!' "

Local hospitals, community colleges, support groups and other organizations offer classes to help you or someone you love stop using drugs. Some cities have drug-use prevention projects for youths.

DRUG-FREE
ZONE
HEALTH & SAFETY CODE 11353.6
A CONVICTION FOR POSSESSION OR THE SALE OF
DRUGS ON OR WITHIN 1000 FT. OF SCHOOL GROUNDS WILL
RESULT IN ADDITIONAL PUNISHMENT.....(A PROLONGED
SENTENCE IN STATE PRISON), AS PROVIDED BY THIS LAW.

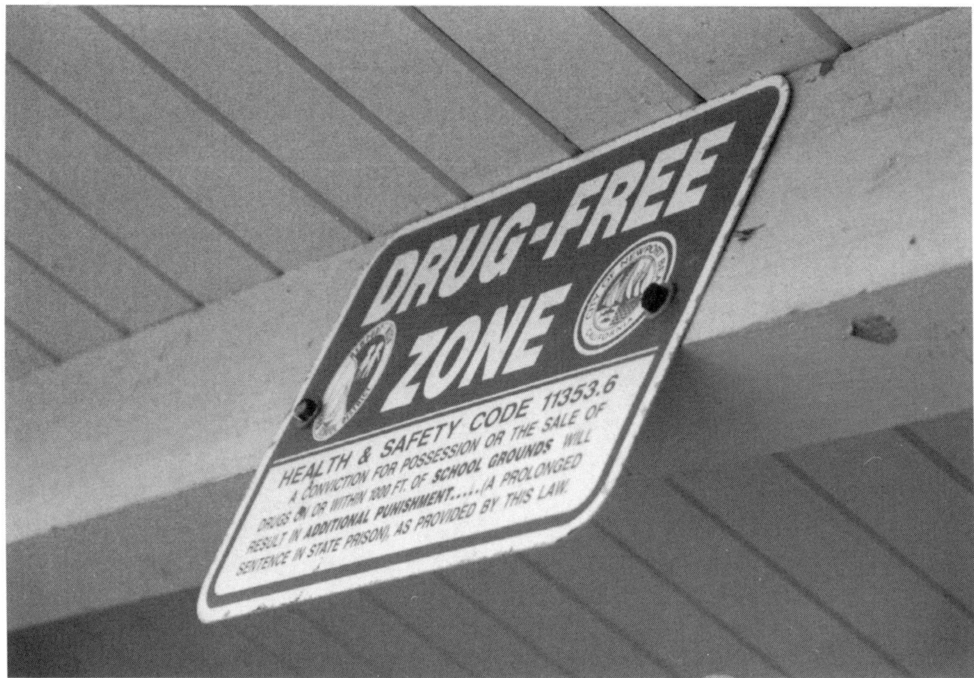

Free, free, free: The Department of Education has a free brochure on growing up drug-free. Call 800-624-0100. The National Crime Prevention Council has a free booklet called, "Don't Lose a Friend to Drugs." Write to 1700 K Street, NW 2nd Floor, Washington, D. C. 20006, or call 800-627-2911. And the American Council for Drug Education will send you free information if you call 800-488-DRUG.

Problems in your family? Check the phone book under Narcotics Anonymous for local numbers.

COME CRAWLING FASTER

"Certain music gives drugs a good reputation. Dogg Pound sings, 'High till I die; don't ask why.' "

Can you name a song, movie scene, ad, commercial or billboard that portrays drugs as glamorous?

____

____

Now, how unreal is that? While some music can glamorize the heavy drug scene, Metallica's song "Master Of Puppets" talks straight:

End of passion play, crumbling away
I'm your source of self-destruction
Veins that pump with fear, sucking darkest clear
Leading on your death's construction

[Chorus:]

Taste me you will see
more is all you need
you're dedicated to
how I'm killing you
Come crawling faster
obey your Master
your life burns faster
obey your Master
Master
Master of Puppets I'm pulling your strings
twisting your mind and smashing your dreams
Blinded by me, you can't see a thing
Just call my name, 'cause I'll hear you scream
Master
Master
Just call my name, 'cause I'll hear you scream
Master
Master

[End Chorus]

Needlework the way, never you betray
life of death becoming clearer
Pain monopoly, ritual misery
chop your breakfast on a mirror

[Chorus]

Master, Master, Where's the dreams that I've been after?
Master, Master, You promised only lies
Laughter, Laughter, All I hear and see is laughter
Laughter, Laughter, laughing at my cries
Hell is worth all that, natural habitat
just a rhyme without a reason
Never-ending maze, drift on numbered days
now your life is out of season

[Chorus]

[Fade out with evil laughter].

KNOCK IT OFF

Whether it's drugs, alcohol, steroids, tobacco or something else that has a grip on you, write down your reasons for quitting. Set a quit date and ask your friends to help you.

Create a commitment form, something like this:

I, ______________________________, promise to stop ________________ as of ______________, [time] on ______________________ [day]. Instead, I will do something other than give in, like relax, exercise, talk, brag, go on a date or__________________ [fill in]. I figure I'll save $________________[big dollar amount] by not paying for self-destruction. I will use that money instead to get __________________ [big dream], which I will get the first week I've cut the strings. But that's not as great as the __________________[bigger dream] I'll get after I've gone 28-days without it. I will NOT give up.

Keep a record of all the days you didn't let your friends pressure you, your cravings get the best of you or your goal vaporize. After 28 days, you'll have established a new, good habit. You'll be free. You can brag a little. Then use the spotlight to help others quit, too.

One Group's Pledge:

"We are banding together to stop this madness so we can have a peaceful and livable home, neighborhood and community."

EATING DISORDERS

"I hid in baggy clothes, threw away my lunches at school and always told my parents I ate dinner at a friend's house. Not eating was like digging myself into a hole."

Eating disorders destroy your body. Starvation screws with your heart, brain and other vital organs. Drugs that stimulate vomiting and going to the bathroom increase your risk of heart failure. Bones, hair and nails become brittle. Skin yellows, dries and wrinkles. Your body temperature drops, as does your ability to handle cold. Your brain shrinks and your sweet, funny personality changes.

Eating disorders tend to run in families. Girls with an eating problem sometimes have mothers who are overly concerned about their daughter's body shape and attractiveness. Fathers and brothers may be overly critical of a girl's weight as well.

"My mother always scolds me to eat less, saying I will never marry if I am overweight. Ever since I was 11, she's been telling me to lose five pounds. Lately, my brother and father have joined in as well. They have this ideal of a Chinese girl as fragile, delicate and thin."

But guys, don't think you're immune. A study by Cornell University found that 40% of its football players had messed-up eating patterns and 10% had outright disorders. Coaches and others say that an athlete who throws up his food to keep his weight down from November to March may find in April that he still wants to do it, even though he doesn't have to "make weight." Throwing up to purge food and release tension is highly addictive.

THREE KINDS OF DISORDERS

1. **Anorexia nervosa:** About 1% of adolescent girls starve themselves. With anorexia, periods stop or become irregular. Consult the Body Mass Index chart on page 99. If you are 15% below acceptable body weight, please listen to your family and friends, and get help now. Don't let your feelings of isolation, disgust or frustration keep you from taking healthy control. Anorexia can kill you. Get help.
2. **Bulimia nervosa:** About 2% to 3% of teen girls develop a destructive pattern of excessive overeating followed by "purging"—throwing up, abusing laxatives or diuretics, taking enemas or obsessively exercising.

Purging may result in heart failure because vital minerals are lost. Vomiting inflames the esophagus and the glands near your cheeks.

Unlike anorexia nervosa sufferers, weight doesn't change much, so it's hard for others to notice your secret. You'll have to get help on your own. Now.

"At my boarding school, so many girls were throwing up their food that by the afternoon, the bathroom just reeked. Most dropped out of school because they couldn't control their urge to purge."

3. **Binge eating:** 2% of Americans—about 1/3 are guys—have uncontrolled episodes of overeating. To reduce stress and relieve anxiety, they stuff themselves, usually with junk food, until they are uncomfortably full. This causes guilt and depression. Most are obese and have a history of weight fluctuations. Binge eating may cause the stomach to rupture. Get help.

SAD STATS

One in 10 cases of all eating disorders lead to death from starvation, cardiac arrest or suicide.

GET HELP NOW

Call a nearby hospital or university medical center to find an eating-disorder clinic near you. Schools, counseling centers and self-help groups listed in the phone book are also good sources.

The National Institutes of Health have a free brochure on eating disorders, available through the Consumer Information Center, Dept. 552C, Pueblo, Colorado 81009 or fax your request to 202-501-4281. Or you can download the information at http://www.pueblo.gsa.gov. Have you memorized that Web address yet? For more information, call 202-501-1794.

The Foundation for Education About Eating Disorders (FEED) can be reached at 410-467-0603.

"I'm a wrestler and the big push is to cut weight, getting down to a specific weight class in wrestling. It can sometimes be a tough and unhealthy experience for wrestlers. I know. I once found myself with a finger down my throat in an attempt to lose weight. Now I know how to lose weight quickly, yet carefully."

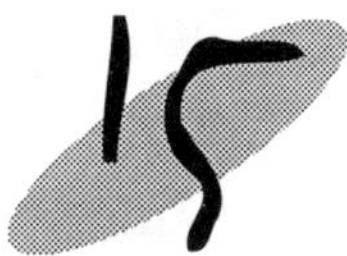

WIGGIN', STRESSIN', DEPRESSIN'

You know it. When you're under stress, your face breaks out, fights break out and bad habits break free. Reduce the tension. How? First, pinpoint the people, places, events and situations that raise the temperature in your life.

Here are some things that drive up your stress thermometer. Check off any of these statements that are generally true about you:

__ My school work is way harsh.

__ I'm always late.

__ I don't like my job.

__ I've got too many responsibilities.

__ I don't have enough fun.

__ I worry about my personal safety.

__ Someone I care about has been ill or has died within the last year.

__ I have a real hard time talking openly to my family or friends.

__ I rarely have time for myself.

__ I feel worn down by the hassles of just living.

__ I'm in a fight with a relative or friend.

__ I'm bummed about my health or weight.

__ I moved out of my family's house.

__ I don't like the way I look.

__ My friends are always trying to get me to join them in taking drugs, drinking alcohol or doing something illegal.

In the space below, list any other major or ongoing causes of stress that are getting to you:

____

____

____

____

TOTAL IMPACT

Now that you've nailed down what causes your stress, look at how you respond. What impact does stress have on your body, brain and behavior? Check out the following list. Circle 0 for **N**ever, 1 for **S**ometimes and 2 for **A**lways.

When I'm under stress, my body lets me know with:

N S A

0 1 2 — headaches
0 1 2 — feeling tired
0 1 2 — waking up in the middle of the night
0 1 2 — upset stomach
0 1 2 — sore back and/or shoulder muscles

When I'm under stress, my behavior changes and I notice I have:

0 1 2 — less ability to work hard
0 1 2 — more irritability and anger
0 1 2 — more eating and snacking
0 1 2 — been smoking, taking drugs or drinking alcohol
0 1 2 — gone wild with spending money
0 1 2 — withdrawn and don't want to be bothered by others
0 1 2 — a change in attitude

When I'm under stress, I notice the following psychological responses:

0 1 2 — I'm sad
0 1 2 — It's hard for me to concentrate
0 1 2 — I feel emotionally drained
0 1 2 — I feel impulsive
0 1 2 — I forget things
0 1 2 — I want to eat more or I don't want to eat
0 1 2 — I feel anxious, short-tempered, edgy

Count up how many points you have. The more 2's you have circled, the more attention you may want to pay to stress in your life, how you manage it and how alternate strategies would be healthier.

YOUR SCORE

30-38: Whoa! You're in orbit. You've got to decompress. You need to get some help.

20-29: You're a rocket on the launch pad with the countdown already started. 10, 9, 8...Push the STOP button. Talk to someone you trust. You're on the edge.

10-19: OK, you've got some problems with stress, but you can handle them. Look out below.

under 10: Really? You've rarely experienced any of these stress-related reactions? Glad to hear it.

"I call exercise my stress buster. It clears my head and puts all my aggression into something positive, instead of fighting with everyone all the time. Sometimes it's heavy running or baseball and other times it's easy-going yoga."

OTHER STRESS BUSTERS

- **Put** on comfy clothes and call a pal. Talk and talk and talk without worrying about the time.
- **Walk** a dog. Pet a cat.
- **Take** a five-minute snooze.
- **Daydream** in a safe place (not behind the wheel of a moving car).
- **Re-read** your favorite poem or book and let yourself enjoy its humor or meaning.
- **Spend** time looking at photographs or videos of people you love.
- **Figure** out a way to create a home, school or work environment that is enjoyable. Talk to a friend or an adult you trust and get solid advice. There is at least one good answer to every question.
- **If** someone is sick and you feel helpless about it, remember that your company means a lot. You can't solve every problem, but you can always be a good friend.
- **Give** yourself enough time to get somewhere. Get up earlier, and don't try to squeeze in more things than you can actually handle. (You may want to pass this advice on to your parents.)
- **Create** time alone for yourself. Maybe listen to your favorite music some place where you won't be interrupted.
- **Fights** usually begin because of a misunderstanding. Someone thinks he or she is not being respected. Don't get mad. Instead, talk openly about how you're feeling. If someone doesn't listen, accept that maybe he or she never will. You don't have to get someone to agree with you 100% to win an argument. State your case and drop it. Give everyone time to think things through and realize the relationship is way more important than a festering disagreement.
- **Rub** the back of your neck and shoulders until you feel more relaxed.
- **Be** careful when it comes to spending. Financial worries can give you big-time headaches. Is having a new car worth going into debt and feeling lousy about it? (Nobody wants to see the repo man at the door.) What if you can't get your clothes out of layaway? Draw up a budget and only buy what you can afford.

◆ **Take** care of business. Get your plan down and work toward it. And don't forget to reward yourself for all the progress you've made.

YEAH, BUT IT'S HEAVIER THAN ALL THAT

Everyone's sad or anxious once in a while—a big test, big date or big challenge can add stress and sometimes disappointment. But if you:

+ can't seem to get motivated about anything,
+ don't want to talk to even your closest friends,
+ feel like nothing you do is fun, exciting or interesting,
+ or you're uptight and short with people, get angry quickly over little things, pushing people away...
= You could be edging toward depression.

Depression is a word bantered around a lot, just like "dysfunctional" and "burnout." But these are words that have real definitions, real heartache and real treatments.

Depression stops you from enjoying life. It's not just feeling down some of the time but feeling sad, worthless, helpless, hopeless, empty, restless, guilty or negative most of the time, for more than two to three weeks. It's a "whole body" illness that affects your body, mood and thoughts—the way you think about yourself and your life.

It can come about because of a serious loss, chronic illness, difficult relationship, financial problem, a move to a new school or an unwanted change in your life. Genetics and psychological factors may play a part as well. Also, taking some drugs—prescribed or otherwise—and drinking alcohol can get you down.

Depression is not your fault. And it isn't because there's a weakness in you. It can't be willed away. You can't just "pull yourself together." Your feelings are changing without your permission. Stuff like:

◆ you're sad a lot
◆ you're no longer the lovable you
◆ you're eating more or less than you used to
◆ you're sleeping more or less than you used to
◆ you don't want to be with people—even friends
◆ you no longer enjoy things that you used to like
◆ you have trouble concentrating, remembering or making decisions
◆ you're dragging
◆ your grades are dropping
◆ you're overly impulsive
◆ you act-out—cover your depression by being angry or aggressive, running away or becoming delinquent
◆ your confidence is gone
◆ you feel like giving up
◆ you have thoughts of death and dying

Get help. Today. You don't have to suffer. A great majority (80%) of people with depression can be treated. Confide in someone: your parents, older siblings, clergy, trusted teacher, or the school psychologist or counselor. Or look in the White Pages in the government section (where the police and fire departments' phone numbers are listed) and find your community's mental health program. It may also be listed in the Yellow Pages under "mental health," "health," "social services," "family service agencies" or "suicide prevention."

If you feel desperate and can't find someone to help, call the police.

HEALTHY HEADS HERE

To maintain a healthy head, take hold of these guidelines, offered by the National Institute of Mental Health:

1. Be realistic. You can't get it all done at once. You can't always have it your way. Slow down and give in a little and you'll find that feeling better takes time...and support from friends.
2. Don't hold back. There aren't good and bad feelings—they're just feelings. Your feelings. Every healthy person feels sadness, anger, frustration, joy, love and satisfaction. Talk about all of these emotions. If you're happy, spread it around. If you're feeling squashed down or ignored, talk it over—calmly, please—with the person who you think is doing it. Don't bottle up or you'll blow up.
3. Get away from it all. Take breaks to feel good, even if you're in the middle of powering through a big report. (Your schedule should always include kick-back time.) Spend time with friends, even if your first impulse is to be alone. Do things that make you feel better (a non-demanding sport? A movie? Watching a ball game?).
4. And while we're on this subject, no sense brooding over something you don't like. Fix it or accept it.
5. Left, right, left, right. One step at a time and you'll make it. Don't take on too much responsibility or set your goals too high. Break big tasks into small ones. If you have to read 210 pages in a week, read 30 pages a day and you won't feel freaked. And set priorities on what's important.
6. Don't blame yourself for not being on top of your game. Do what you can. Then stop and enjoy what you accomplished.
7. Don't listen to negative thinking. It's part of depression. Take control of your brain's keyboard and rewrite what's on the screen.
8. Lean on your family and friends. Tell them what you're going through (explain what depression is) and ask them to be understanding, patient, affectionate and encouraging. Get someone to listen.

For more information, write to D/ART Public Inquiries, National Institute of Mental Health, Room 7C-02, 5600 Fishers Lane, Rockville, MD 20857 or call 800-421-4211.

FEELING DESPERATE

As much as we'd like to ignore it, suicide is a reality. It's the ultimate response to unbearable pain. Someone who's feeling so low that death seems like a step up—though it never is—may attempt to hurt him or herself.

If you know someone who is feeling depressed and desperate, who thinks everything is going wrong, please listen to him or her carefully. Your friend may be asking for help.

Maybe his life has been spun around or she's being abused or neglected. Maybe someone close to him has recently died or moved away. Maybe he suffers from learning disabilities or feels alone. Maybe she's a perfectionist who was devastated when her performance slipped. Maybe he's aggressive or anxious.

If you or your friend is:

- **withdrawing** from friends;
- **feeling** isolated or rejected;
- **being** disruptive, running away, acting violent, crying easily;
- **neglecting** his or her looks;
- **thinking** about death all the time;
- **writing** poems or journal entries about death;
- **listening** to music that glorifies suicide or dancing the "suicide" (an aerial flip that finishes with a body slam);
- **saying** things like, "You'll be better off when I'm gone";
- **giving** away favorite things;
- **changing** eating or sleeping habits;
- **abusing** alcohol or drugs;
- **constantly** feeling pushed to reach a high level of success and status;
- **feeling** overwhelmed by outside pressures—academic competition, drugs, the push to have sex, to fit in;
- **playing** with weapons;
- **or** doing anything that worries you, ***please take these steps*:**

1. Talk to an adult. Tell them what's going on. Ask them to help you.

"It's better that my friend gets mad at me for telling someone than for my friend to be dead."

---

2. Watch out for guns. People who are in homes with firearms are five times more likely to kill themselves than those who don't have access to them.
3. If you or your friend can't talk to your parents, talk to someone. Some schools offer anti-suicide classes. Information is always good. Talking openly about a problem with someone you trust helps us to better understand what it is and find ways to solve the problem.

"Whatever the problem is, we can work it out."

---

4. If you don't feel comfortable talking to someone in person, call one of these hotlines and ask for help. That's why they're there:
   - **Teen** Line: 800-TLC-TEEN
   - **The** Suicide Prevention Center Crisis Line in your area (in Los Angeles, for example, it's 310-391-1253). Call 411 for the local number.
   - **Youth** Crisis Hotline: 800-HIT-HOME or 800-442-HOPE.
   - **National** Runaway Switchboard: 800-621-4000

"I think of Kurt Cobain who wrote, 'You can't fire me. I quit.' And I think, what a waste that he's dead. He said a lot of important things and the world still needs him. Everyone has more things to come into their life and if they end it now, how will they get to the good stuff that is going to happen in the future?"

Part 3

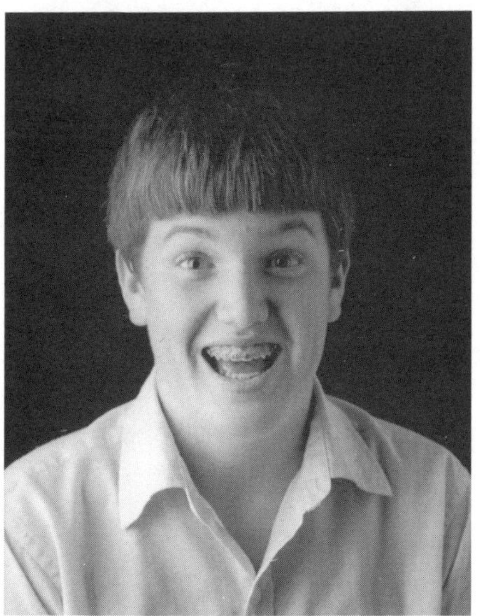

DROPPING POUNDAGE

In this section, you'll learn how to follow a safe, proven weight-loss program. You'll be eating real food available everywhere, even in grease pits. And you won't feel deprived or like an outsider.

SO YOU NEED TO LOSE

Ask a girl, any girl, how much she weighs. "Go ahead," goads Michelle, a high school senior. "I dare you. If you're lucky, she won't slap you, melt you with a withering glare or pretend you don't exist. If you're really lucky, she might even give you an answer.

"Then all you have to do is add about 10 pounds, divide her waistline by her height, subtract that by her age, then multiply that by the number of chocolate chip cookies she ate that day. And you might come reasonably close to her true weight."

It's not that teen girls lie about how much they weigh. Some couldn't care less about what the bathroom scale reveals. Others are afraid to look at the numbers and just assume the worst. Many times they've overestimated their weight. But then there are girls like Michelle who know down to the ounce what they tip the scale at...that's where the creativity begins.

Michelle admits, "Even the most honest among us have no qualms about subtracting a few pounds from our actual weight because that's how much we will weigh in a few weeks once we go on the diet that begins tomorrow."

LESSON ONE

How to be a typical junior high school girl:

In the bathroom, step out of the stall. Two of your friends are waiting for you (the rule is that girls never travel alone). As you wash your hands in the sink, look in the mirror and lament, "I am so fat."

To this, the first friend will protest, "Whatever! You're a little toothpick. I'm the fat one."

"No, look at me!" friend Number Two will cry. "I need to lose at least 10 pounds." You're laughing? In high school, it doesn't get much better.

LESSON TWO

How to be a typical high school girl:

At lunch time, the trendy thing to do is only order a salad and a diet soda. Then take two-and-a-half bites of lettuce, throw down your fork and pronounce how you are such a pig and so full that you just can't stuff another bite down your throat. In doing this, you'll succeed in making the other girls at the table shove aside their plates in guilt.

Sound familiar? Well, not to the boys. Can you imagine guys talking about feeling bloated? Staying up all night at a sleepover yakking about how they wished they looked like models? "Oh, that guy in GQ is so awesome!" Right. Can you picture boys spending hours in front of a full-length mirror picking apart and hating their bodies?

It's hard to imagine. What's the difference between boys and girls beside the obvious stuff? Boys rarely talk about how much they weigh unless it's something they need to be aware of because of a weight-classification for a sport like wrestling or boxing or if they're actually proud of their size.

These two worlds stay divided into adulthood. Surveys show that most women interviewed think they need to lose pounds even when they are at a healthy weight, while many men who are overweight think they are at least close to where they should be.

So, what does it take to get a guy thinking that maybe he's on the hefty side? Insults. Jabs. Cruel comments. Rude remarks. Put downs. Verbal slaps and pokes. Slurs. Zingers. Or maybe a helpful talk by his doctor.

"Kids make fun of me at school, but I really don't care," says Nam, a freshman. "Other boys would run up to me, pull at my chest and yell, `fat titties.' In the 4th grade, it bothered me, but now I just laugh back at them. It's the best way to take it because if they think it doesn't hurt you, then they'll stop. A kid who weighs five pounds less than me—he eats a lot of fried chicken every day—gets it now from the other kids."

There are a lot of bummers about being overweight. You know, the mean talk hurled at the fat teens. Aimee was called Shamu. Mike would hear, "Look at the fat kid loser." Stas was never picked to be on a team because guys would say, "He's so fat, he can't run."

"If kids are teased too much or are always treated as the scapegoat ("George did it"), they can become depressed. They can act like wallflowers or do the opposite, be bullies who are mean and nasty to other kids because they feel bad about themselves."

Nam thought he was doing a good job of blocking out the insults, then something happened that made him realize he couldn't ignore the fact that he was overweight.

When he went to get a physical to enter high school, the nurse told him he was 5' 6" and weighed 211 pounds. "I weighed myself about a month ago and I was 180," he said. "I thought I was 180."

Nam kept repeating the same words: "I thought I was 180." This happens a lot. Teens think they're cruising along and, suddenly, reality hits. Even XXL T-shirts hug around the middle. People start hinting that maybe some pounds should be dropped. A reflection in the mirror becomes a troubling image.

"The other day I was walking with my thin friends and noticed that of our shadows in front of me, mine was twice as large."

Nam wants to lose weight. "People tell me I'll outgrow it, but if I stay exactly the same weight I am now, I'll have to grow to be 6′5"—as tall as a pro basketball player—to even out the score."

Yeah, you're right Nam. You need a plan. Exercise is part of it, but exercise alone won't do it if you're slopping butter onto everything. You have to change the way you eat, as do one out of every three of your friends who is packing 15 to 20 pounds more than what's healthy.

WHY LOSE?

It may make you uncomfortable to read this part, but it may also help you see that being fat hurts. Not just your feelings, but your body.

- **20%** to 30% of 3- to 18-year olds have above average total cholesterol levels and decreased amounts of "good" high-density lipoprotein (HDL) cholesterol, says the American Health Foundation. Overweight teens also have higher blood pressure levels.
- **As** early as 3, kids can develop fatty streaks—deposits in blood vessels that lead to clogged arteries and heart attacks as adults.

"If you eat junk food and few proteins and nutrients, you will be shorter. I read that somewhere or maybe my doctor told me."

- **Another** depressing fact: The American Heart Association says there has been a 54% jump in obesity in American kids since 1969.

TATER TOT TODAY, COUCH POTATO TOMORROW

If you're overweight now, it's likely you'll grow up to be a heavy adult. "The longer you remain overweight, the greater the likelihood that the problem will persist into adulthood," says Dr. Ronald Kleinman of the Committee on Nutrition of the American Academy of Pediatrics.

Unless you change now.

A government study followed the medical histories of 508 people from childhood to age 70. It discovered that fat teenage boys are more likely to be overweight men who have heart problems, colon cancer and an 80% higher risk of premature death, compared to men who were fit most of their lives.

Overly chubby teen girls will likely become overweight women who have arthritis, heart disease and other problems. By age 70, these women will find it harder than fit senior citizens to take a walk more than a block, lift objects heavier than a few pounds or climb stairs.

WHY ARE KIDS FATTER TODAY?

Simple. They eat too much junk food and their bodies lie motionless, or close to it, too many hours every day. There's not as much chance to run around at school; many schools have axed PE programs because there's not enough money or equipment. Fewer than one-third of schools offer PE classes where you're supposed to be taught a lifelong fitness program.

When you're out of school, all your time is eaten up doing things other than sweating for fun.

"If you go to a park, you'll find the adults are running and the kids aren't. Too many teens move slow, they don't do anything. They veg."

Pollution, crime and other environmental factors sometimes make it unsafe to play outside. So what do you do? Slop down inside and spend your time watching TV, maneuvering video games, talking on the phone, hanging up posters, driving your family crazy with your opinions? All are worth exploring, but not at the cost of exercise and your health. You want to be around for a long time so you can see all those ideas your family thinks will never work Bill-Gates the world.

Speaking of the world, how do American teens compare physically to teens living in other parts of the world? A decade's worth of fitness tests and medical studies show that teens in the U.S. are generally heavier, less active and less interested in physical activity than France's *adolescentes* , Korea's *chung nyun*, Spain's *pijos*, Japan's *judai* or Mexico's *jovenes*.

THINK YOU'RE READY?

If you need to drop some pounds, you've come to the right place. But not everyone needs to lose weight. First, really look at yourself in the mirror and see if there's excess to lose. For most, it's more a matter of firming up through exercise than dieting.

Want to know which category you're in?

Take this simple test: It's called a BMI. No, it's not an expensive German sports car. It's about your Body Mass Index.

Researchers who think about obesity and weight all day long use this figure to measure bigness (they call it "ponderosity" because big words turn them on). The number is based on your gender, weight and height and will show you if you're healthy, underweight or overweight.

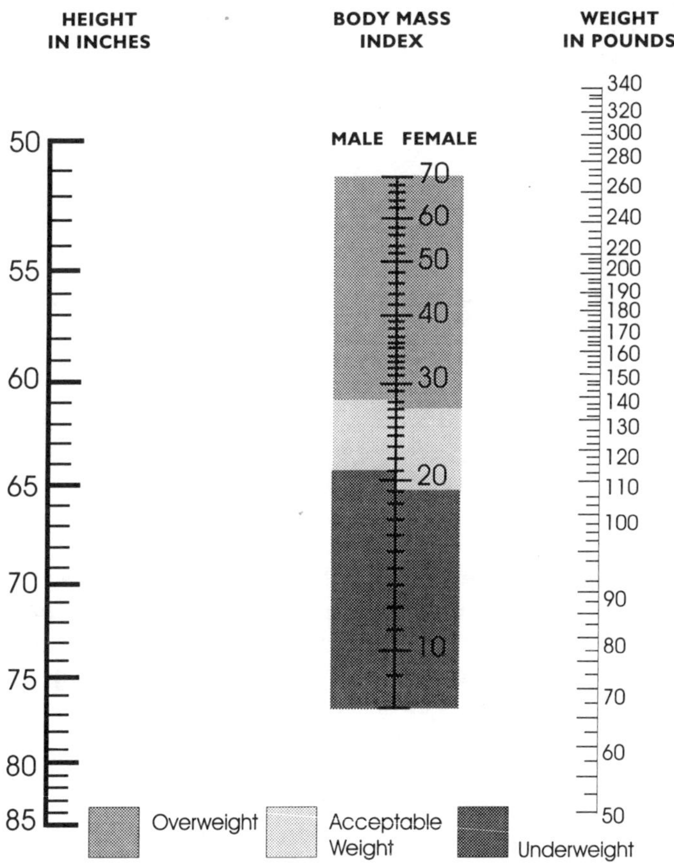

To determine your BMI, draw a line from your height (on the left side of the illustration) to your weight (on the right). Your BMI is the number at which that line crosses the center. The healthy BMI range is in the shaded zone.

If your BMI is in the shaded zone (the acceptable weight range) or dark gray zone (the underweight range), don't even think about dieting. You don't need it. Reread Chapter 6 on positive self image, take a walk and relax.

If your BMI is in the light gray zone, you're at risk of being overweight. Talk to your parents about this book and see if losing weight is something you all can work on together.

You may also benefit from a medical diagnosis. Bring this book with you and have your doctor review the menu. Tell the doctor and your parents—and anyone else who will listen—that in the weight-loss part of *bodyPRIDE*:

- **you'll** learn about your body's chemistry and how it fuels itself.
- **you'll** eat real foods.
- **you** won't feel hungry or deprived.
- **you'll** forget about counting calories. Instead, you'll see what kinds of foods burn stored fat.

And you'll do it day by day, beginning with:

PREP DAY ONE

> "Prep days are awesome. The best days of your life. You'll like it. You get to eat....Well, you'll see."

For the first three days, you'll be beefing up your body and getting it ready to lose weight by eating foods higher in fat, oils and proteins. It's kinda like filling up your car before you go on a trip.

For these three days you may shovel down some fried shrimp, fried chicken, onion rings, fried zucchini sticks, whipped cream, whole milk and vegetable oils if you want to get those munchies out of your system. If this seems like your regular menu, these three prep days may not be necessary because you already have a healthy reserve of essential fatty acids and amino acids. But if you've been cutting back recently, use these three prep days to boost up your body. This will encourage normal gallbladder activity and help to protect you against the development of gallstones, those painful, cholesterol balls blocking bile (ugh, hurts me).

GIVE IT TO ME AGAIN

This means that for three days you can chow down not just a cheeseburger but a BACON cheeseburger. Not just a salad with gooey dressing but a chef salad with ham and bacon and a spoonful of fatty, creamy dressings (Caesar, anyone?). Not just a Grand Slam breakfast with eggs, sausage and greasy hash browns, but....you get the idea.

Ugh. One thing, though. Don't binge eat. This isn't a grand pigout. Barfing is totally discouraged. Also, you can't eat candy, cakes, pies, cookies, sugary gum, breads—doughy stuff —and as always, no alcohol. But who needs sugar when a mountain of buttery mashed potatoes is in front of you and everyone around you is saying, "Dig in!"

Fruits and vegetables will never hurt you, so indulge every day of your life. During the three prep days, add peanut butter to your celery or apple slices, and butter to your veggies.

Don't worry if you gain a few pounds—those will drop off within the first days of the diet. Also, you may experience a minor, temporary increase in your blood cholesterol level, but that will be corrected, too. During the diet you should have a healthy decrease of bad cholesterol as well as improved HDL (the "good cholesterol").

Also, water is your friend. Glug 64 ounces throughout the day to keep you afloat. If it seems hard at first to swallow that much, build up each day to the big 64. After awhile, your body will crave it and it'll be easier. Hey, and don't forget your vitamins. Your DAP is waiting to be written all over.

BRING IT ON

Here's an example of a Prep Day Menu:

Breakfast

2 fried eggs
2 strips of bacon or sausage
1 slice of whole wheat toast with butter
6 to 8 oz. orange juice

Lunch

Cheeseburger, hot dog or pizza with everything
French fries
Fresh fruit
Salad with creamy dressing
Diet soda

Dinner

6 ounces of steak, pork chops, ham, lamb or a serving of gooey Fettuccine Alfredo
Baked potato with butter and sour cream
Salad with creamy dressing

Snacks

Nuts, seeds, cheese

ANY THOUGHTS BEFORE YOU TAKE OFF?

______

______

______

______

______

______

PREP DAY ONE

DAILY ACTION PLAN

• Day

• Date

• BREAKFAST

Healthy snack

• LUNCH

Healthy snack

• DINNER

Occasional Dessert

How Many Carbs?

How Much Fat?

Vitamins?

Yep! Nope.

How much Water?

Weight?

How Many Steps?

• For Exercise, I

• I Am Great because

• My Dream is

• To reach it, today I will

• If happens, I will

• My reward today is

O.K. So Instead I'm On www.bodypride.com

PREP DAY TWO

(Yes, just keep eating away at those high-fat options suggested in Prep Day One).

The first day of your weight-loss phase of the program is just two days away. Before you start, ask yourself an important question: "How much weight do I need to lose?"

You do the math:

Write in your current weight: _________pounds

Subtract your BMI weight* (see page 99): _________pounds

This is your weight-loss goal: _________pounds

[*Since you're still growing vertically, we suggest you aim for the highest weight in the acceptable weight range on the BMI chart. If the range is 140 to 155 pounds, your goal weight should be 155 pounds.]

For example, Jenn is 5′6″ and weighs 160. She looks at the BMI chart and sees the range for girls who are 5′6″ is 115 to 150 pounds. She fills out her goal-weight wish list this way:

Write in your current weight: 160 pounds

Subtract your BMI weight*: (see page 99): 150 pounds

This is your weight-loss goal: 10 pounds

In Jenn's case, her weight-loss goal is 10 pounds.

Now's a good time to wrap a tape measure around parts of your body. Measure your:

- height _______
- chest _______
- waist _______
- lower abdomen _______
- hips _______
- and upper thigh _______

Jot down the numbers here. This is good to do every week or so to chart your progress.

PREP DAY TWO

DAILY ACTION PLAN

• Day ....

• Date ....

• BREAKFAST ....

Healthy snack ....

• LUNCH ....

Healthy snack ....

• DINNER ....

Occasional Dessert ....

How Many Carbs? [ ] How Much Fat? [ ]

Vitamins? [ ] Yep! [ ] Nope.

How much Water? [ ]

Weight? [ ]

How Many Steps? [ ]

• For Exercise, I ....

• I Am Great because ....

• My Dream is ....

• To reach it, today I will ....

• If .... happens, I will ....

• My reward today is ....

O.K. So Instead I'm On www.bodypride.com

PREP DAY THREE

How does that pizza taste? Well, enjoy it on this, the last prep day. It won't taste quite the same to you once you realize how it works over your body.

Today is also a great day to run, run, run. Or walk, walk, walk. Or do whatever you like to do to move your bones and muscles. Any kind of movement you do will make weight loss easier and faster. And you'll stick to it if you find an activity you love and do it three to four days a week for 20 minutes. A step counter will record most of your movements. If you're on a bike, clip it to your shoe to make sure you score a step for every time you push the pedal.

TAKE A CHANCE

No matter how enthusiastic you are when you start the program, it's easy to lose oomph once the initial excitement fades. That's why it helps to have a visual reminder of your goals.

Here's an idea: why not create an "after" photograph of yourself? Get two pictures of yourself in a swimsuit or shorts. Use one as a "before" picture. With the other, take a pen and outline a leaner, healthier body shape. Use scissors to trim away the weight you're determined to lose. It's your future. Picture it.

YOUR SPACE

PREP DAY THREE

DAILY ACTION PLAN

- Day ....
- Date ....

- BREAKFAST ....
  - Healthy snack ....
- LUNCH ....
  - Healthy snack ....
- DINNER ....
  - Occasional Dessert ....

How Many Carbs? | How Much Fat?

Vitamins? ☐ Yep! ☐ Nope.

How much Water?

Weight?

How Many Steps?

- For Exercise, I ....
- I Am Great because ....
- My Dream is ....
- To reach it, today I will ....
- If .... happens, I will ....
- My reward today is ....

O.K. So Instead I'm On www.bodypride.com

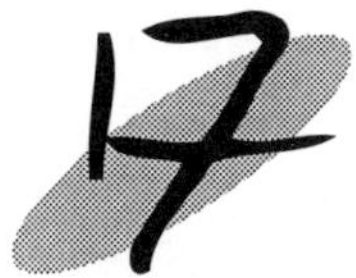

WHY DIETS ARE DRAGS

Maybe you've been on a diet before and it failed to work You probably hated that it was a hard-nosed program that forced you to give up everything you love, like gooey, sweet things. Pretty soon, you were feeling like a machine that does everything it's programmed to do. Maybe that bugged you and you went off and ate something forbidden.

Two hits came with that: You felt like a cheater who deserved to be fat. You then felt so bad that you stuffed yourself to the breaking point. Yikes! That wrong move put back on every pound you'd lost before...and maybe more. Making matters worse, your family and friends thought you didn't try hard enough. You felt out of control.

THAT'S NOT TRUE

You're in control. And you know that everything you do has a grand purpose. You deserve to feel better, especially about yourself.

That's what this weight-loss program is all about. We're not gonna beat you up and point out your failures. If you have a temporary setback, relax. You can start up again and regain the momentum.

BUT FIRST STEPS...

First, you're going to change your body from a fat-storage bin to a fat-burning machine. You'll do that by following this safe, nutritious and easy-to-understand menu for 28 days. It gives you high-protein, low-calorie, low-carb choices—real food—that will jump-start your body into becoming a PacMan gobbling up stored fat.

When your body burns fat stores, it converts it into ketone bodies. Just like when you burn a fire and ashes are left in the fireplace, when fat is burned, invisible ketones are left over. Your body uses these ketones for energy. It's like high-octane fuel. The leftover ketone bodies are dumped out through your urine.

If you're the scientific type who wants to verify what's happening in your body, you can do this by peeing on a ketostick, a stick that changes to a lavender color when enough ketones are present. Ketosticks are sold at pharmacies. Every morning, walk into the bathroon, do your thing, and pass the ketostick through your urine stream. If you're burning a lot of fat, your urine will have enough ketones to turn the ketostick color. That's called being in a state of "ketosis." You've become a fat-burning machine!

The benefit of being in mild ketosis is that you'll burn excess body fat safely and rapidly while keeping your lean muscle mass. You'll have fewer cravings and be less hungry, less often than with other diets. And since this is all natural, you'll experience more energy and feel terrific.

The drawback? Well, you're not going to like this, but do you like being overweight? Didn't think so. Anyway, ketones come out in your breath as well as your urine, and you may have bad breath. Brushing regularly and chewing sugar-free gum or calorie-free breath fresheners will take care of that. (The reward? You'll know the program's working. Teens tell us they really like this instant feedback.)

***Important:* A ketogenic program is not recommended if you're pregnant or nursing, have a serious liver or kidney disease, or if you're a Type 1, insulin-dependent diabetic. If you're unsure whether this program will be good for you, check with your health-care professional.**

TAH-DAH! THE COMPLETE MENU

"I thought it would be like, 'ok, you little punk. Here's the deal. You're going on a diet. You're gonna be eating wood and bricks. Now shut up!'"

Fooled you.

Breakfast

1 meat/protein
1 fruit *or* 1 grain
Choice of any calorie-free beverage

Morning Snack

Choice of one serving from the protein list

Lunch

1 meat/protein
1 vegetable
1 fruit
2 cups torn lettuce
Salad dressing (choice of any nonfat product, up to 15 calories and 3 grams carbohydrate)
Choice of any calorie free-beverage

Afternoon Snack

Choice of one serving from the Protein list.

Dinner

1 meat/protein
1 vegetable
1 fruit
2 cups torn lettuce
Salad dressing (choice of any nonfat product, up to 15 calories and 3 grams carbohydrate)
Choice of any calorie-free beverage

Evening Snack

Choice of one serving from the Protein list.

FOOD CHOICES, SERVINGS AND CARBOHYDRATE COUNTS

Grains

Your breakfast menu includes your choice of either one serving of fruit *or* one serving of grain from the following list:

Food Choice	Serving	Usable Carbohydrates Per Serving	Food Choice	Serving	Usable Carbohydrates Per Serving
Bread (whole grain, 70 calories or less)	1 slice	13	Nutri-Grain (Barley)	3/4 cup	26
			(Corn)	"	27
Cheerios	3/4 cup	12	Nutri-Grain (Rye)	3/4 cup	25
Chex (Bran)	"	30	(Wheat)	"	28
(Corn)	"	19	Oatmeal (cooked)	1/2 cup	12
(Rice)	"	19			
(Wheat)	"	28	Post Oat Flakes	3/4 cup	21
Cream of Wheat (cooked)	1/2 cup	13	Post Bran Flakes	"	23
			Product 19	"	21
Cream of Rice	"	14	Rice Krispies	3/4 cup	18
Crispix	3/4 cup	19	Shredded Wheat (or Wheat Bran)	"	23
Grapenut Flakes	"	17			
Kashi (Puffed)	"	12	Special K	"	16
Kellogg's 40+ (Bran Flakes)	"	23	Team Flakes	"	27
			Toasties	"	18
Life	"	24	Total (Wheat)	"	17
Malt-O-Meal (cooked)	1/2 cup	13	(Corn)	"	18
			Wheaties	"	18

Protein

Your choice of one serving each at ***breakfast, morning snack, lunch, afternoon snack, dinner***, and ***evening snack***. Be sure to weigh meat, seafood, and poultry (raw, skinned and boned), with all visible fat removed. Broil, boil, barbecue, microwave, roast, or "fry" in a nonstick pan using Pam spray or an equivalent nonfat, nonstick spray.

Food Choice	Serving	Usable Carbohydrates Per Serving	Food Choice	Serving	Usable Carbohydrates Per Serving
Meat and Poultry			(ground)		
Beef heart	3-1/2 oz.	3	Beef flank	3-1/2 oz.	0
			Beef round	"	0

Food Choice	Serving	Usable Carbohydrates Per Serving	Food Choice	Serving	Usable Carbohydrates Per Serving
Chicken breast (fresh or frozen)	"	0	Salmon	"	0
			Scallops	"	2
Chicken breast (canned white, water-packed)	2-1/2 oz.	0	Sea Bass	"	0
			Shark	"	0
			Shrimp	"	1
Cold cuts (97-98% lean/fat free)	2-1/2 oz.	1	Snapper	"	0
			Sole	"	0
Turkey (white breast)	3-1/2 oz.	0	Swordfish	"	0
Veal	3-1/2 oz.	0	Trout (Rainbow)	"	0
Vegetarian			Tuna (white, fresh or frozen)	"	0
Tofu	4 oz	2			
Veg-e-burger	1/3 cup	3			
Veg-e-cutlet or meat substitute	No less than 15 grams of protein per serving	No more 12 grams of carbohydrate per serving	Tuna (canned white albacore, water-packed)	2-1/2 oz.	0
			Turbot	3-1/2 oz.	0
Seafood			**Dairy**		
Catfish	3-1/2 oz.	0	Cheese (fat-free)	2 oz.	0
Cod	"	0	Cottage cheese (lowfat, plain)	4 oz.	4
Crab	"	1			
Haddock	"	0	Egg (limit if cholesterol is high or use EggBeaters)	1	1
Halibut	"	0			
Lobster	"	1			
Orange roughy	"	0	Milk (nonfat)	1 cup	12
Perch	"	0	Yogurt (nonfat, plain)	1/2 cup	9

Vegetables

Your choice of one serving each at ***lunch*** and ***dinner***. Measure raw, frozen (thawed), water packed (drained), unless otherwise stated. No sugar added.

Food Choice	Serving	Usable Carbohydrates Per Serving	Food Choice	Serving	Usable Carbohydrates Per Serving
Asparagus	1 cup	8	Mushrooms, raw	2 cups	7
Bean sprouts	"	14	Okra	1 cup	8
Broccoli	"	5	Onion	1/2 cup	6
Cabbage	"	4	Pepper (red or green)	1 small	4
Carrots	1/2 cup	8			
Celery	1 cup	6	Spinach (raw)	2 cups	4
Chinese pea pods	"	11	(cooked)	1 cup	7
Cauliflower	"	5	String beans	"	8
Collard greens	1 cup	8	Sauerkraut	"	10
Cucumbers	"	3	Tomato	1 small	5
Jicama	1/2 cup	5	Zucchini	1 cup	4

Fruits

Your choice of one serving each at ***breakfast*** (when not choosing a grain), ***lunch*** and ***dinner***. Be sure your daily fruit choices include at least one citrus (indicated with a *). Choose fresh, frozen (thawed), or water packed (without sugar or fruit juice).

Food Choice	Serving	Usable Carbohydrates Per Serving
Apple	1, 2-1/2" dia.	17
Applesauce (unsweetened)	1/2 cup	14
Apricots (fresh)	2 medium	9
(dried)	4 halves	9
Banana	1/2 small	13
Blackberries	2/3 cup	12
Blueberries	"	14
Boysenberries	"	11
Casaba melon	1/4 (6-1/2" dia.)	4
Cantaloupe	1/4 (6" dia.)	11
Cherries	10	11
Dates	2	13
Grapefruit*	1/2 small	10
Grapefruit juice*	4 oz.	11

Food Choice	Serving	Usable Carbohydrates Per Serving
Honeydew melon	1/6 (6-1/2" dia)	20
Orange*	1 small	14
Orange juice* (unsweetened)	4 oz.	12
Papaya	1/2 cup, cubed	7
Peach	1 small	10
Pear (Bartlett)	1/2 small	13
Persimmon	1	8
Pineapple	1/2 cup, cubed	10
Raisins	1/2 oz.	11
Raspberries	2/3 cup	10
Rhubarb	1 cup	7
Strawberries	1 cup	11
Tangerine*	1 (2-1/2" dia.)	9
Watermelon	1/2 cup, cubed	6

Miscellaneous

Your choice of one serving, twice per day, with the meals of your choice.

Food Choice	Serving	Usable Carbohydrates Per Serving
Gelatin (diet)	1/2 cup	0
Green onion (tops)	1 tsp.	0
Horseradish	"	1
Margarine (nonfat, 5 cal max.)	1 Tbs.	0

Food Choice	Serving	Usable Carbohydrates Per Serving
Mustard	1 tsp.	0
Peppers, jalapeño	2 small	2
Pimento	"	1
Radishes	2 medium	1
Vinegar (unseasoned)	2 Tbs.	2

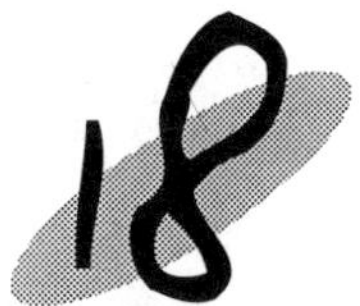

I'M WAITING

You're a mad scientist who experiments every day with this test tube called your body. You add chemicals and minerals and nutrients to it, and watch it grow, expand or explode. It's a chemistry that is uniquely you.

Of all the foods you can eat, your body likes burning carbohydrates the best. Your brain winks happily and says, "thanks very much for the fuel," whenever you chow down on junk food, sugar or starches. If you feed yourself a lot of carbs, your body burns that fresh fuel and stores leftover fuel as fat. But if you eat proteins and limit your carbs and calories, you'll burn that old fuel—the stored fat you're holding in your stomach, thighs and arms.

DAY ONE

Starting today and for the next four weeks, you'll eat about 100 grams of protein—like egg whites, tuna, turkey breast, tofu—and limit your carb intake to between 80 and 100 grams, choosing from the list of fruits, vegetables and grains. This will start you on your way to burning stored body fat while strengthening your lean mass—your bones, muscles, organs and other stuff you need to not flop around like a Slinky curling down the stairs.

Pick your favorite choices from the menu for your meals today and record them on your DAP (you'll find one for every day you're on the plan). Amazing but true: People who complete their DAPs every day have the best results.

YOUR SPACE

DAY ONE

DAILY ACTION PLAN

• Day

• Date

• BREAKFAST

Healthy snack

• LUNCH

Healthy snack

• DINNER

Occasional Dessert

How Many Carbs?

How Much Fat?

Vitamins?

☐ Yep! ☐ Nope.

How much Water?

Weight?

How Many Steps?

• For Exercise, I

• I Am Great because

• My Dream is

• To reach it, today I will

• If happens, I will

• My reward today is

O.K. So Instead I'm On www.bodypride.com

DAY TWO

Did you enjoy yesterday's feast? Well, you get to have another one. Eat your proteins today and limit your carbs to 80 to 100 grams. (Hint: Make it easy on yourself. Pick your favorite foods from the menu so you enjoy what you're eating).

HOW MUCH, HOW FAST?

The amount you lose on this diet depends on your age, gender, starting weight, level of exercise or other activity, and how carefully you follow the program. Most teens safely lose two to five pounds a week.

HEY, DON'T FORGET YOUR FRIEND, DAP

The food diary part of your Daily Action Plan will help you keep track of everything you put in your mouth. Fill it out after every meal, because if you wait hours—or days—you'll forget (your mind is full of more important things than food).

If you gain weight at any time in the future, refer to your food diary and you'll be able to figure out what may have triggered it (maybe you ate too many starchy or fatty foods...or maybe you grew. When you shoot up, go back to the BMI index on page 99 and reconfigure your goal weight. Remember, always shoot for the highest number in the weight range).

Or maybe you lost weight when you didn't want to. Unintentional weight loss could be because you're not eating enough. Less is not best. Stick to the menu and don't skip. You're not helping your body by starving yourself (read Chapter 3 on the importance of three good meals a day).

Your DAP also has space for your exercise heroics. Weight gain could be because your cousin The Slug visited over the weekend and you vegged out with her. Get moving again.

And one thing about your bathroom scale: It is not a judge or jury that decides your value as a person. It just measures your weight. *Nada mas.*

YOUR SPACE

DAY TWO

DAILY ACTION PLAN

• Day ....

• Date ....

• BREAKFAST ....

....

Healthy snack ....

....

• LUNCH ....

....

Healthy snack ....

....

• DINNER ....

....

Occasional Dessert ....

How Many Carbs? [ ] How Much Fat? [ ]

Vitamins? [ ] Yep! [ ] Nope.

How much Water? [ ]

Weight? [ ]

How Many Steps? [ ]

• For Exercise, I ....

....

• I Am Great because ....

....

• My Dream is ....

....

• To reach it, today I will ....

....

• If .... happens, I will ....

....

• My reward today is ....

O.K. So Instead I'm On www.bodypride.com

DAY THREE

The number one reason people stop a diet? Surveys say they don't feel well. You're eating three complete meals a day and you feel great, right? Remember, this is all part of the big plan. We're working on building better bodies and better bodies are bodies that feel good.

HOW'D THEY GET THERE?

It takes a few days to change your body chemistry from being a carb-craver to a ketone-maker. By now, you should be showing some color on your ketostick. If not, you accidentally ate too many carbs. That's easy to do because carbs are hidden in cough syrup, Sweet 'n Low and other stuff. Read the label on everything. Carbs are really sneaky, like your kid sister or brother.

MY HEAD IS SPINNING

Every now and then some people have a giddy reaction when they go on a diet. They feel a little lightheaded and different. If this happens to you, don't freak. This is normal. In fact, you might want to expect it. It comes with a change in your diet and it won't hurt you, if you're following your plan carefully.

You may go through a sugar or carb withdrawal, leaving you feeling a little draggy. While this sounds like a good reason to stay home sick from school all during finals week, don't add more problems and stresses on yourself. Let your parents know that it's a natural reaction whenever you make significant changes in your diet. Your vitamins help here.

Also, some people get less salt when they change their diet. If you feel dizzy when you stand up, add some salt to your food to restore your sodium level (this doesn't mean tunneling through a bag of chips or sucking on the salt shaker). Sprinkle 1/8th of a teaspoon of salt on your protein choice to restore your sodium level.

One other thing to remember: Don't *ever* ignore your body's call for help. Respond to it right away by talking to your parents and re-reading this section on how to combat those temporary, uncomfortable feelings. And jump to our Web site at **www.bodypride.com** for answers to the most common questions. We're here to help.

YOUR SPACE

DAY THREE

DAILY ACTION PLAN

• Day ....

• Date ....

• BREAKFAST ....

....

Healthy snack ....

....

• LUNCH ....

....

Healthy snack ....

....

• DINNER ....

....

Occasional Dessert ....

How Many Carbs? How Much Fat?

Vitamins?

☐ Yep! ☐ Nope.

How much Water?

Weight?

How Many Steps?

• For Exercise, I ....

....

• I Am Great because ....

....

• My Dream is ....

....

• To reach it, today I will ....

....

• If .... happens, I will ....

....

• My reward today is ....

O.K. So Instead I'm On www.bodypride.com

DAY FOUR

You're following the healthy menu and you're dropping ketones like fleas from a shaggy dog. OK, maybe that's not the image you're after.

Final reminder: Eat breakfast foods at breakfast, lunch foods at lunch and dinner foods at dinner. Sound obvious? You bet. But somewhere along the way you may wonder, "May I have my grain at dinner?" and you'll have to read this again: Eat breakfast foods at breakfast, lunch foods at lunch and dinner foods at dinner.

BBQ FOR YOU

Weigh meat, seafood and poultry raw, skinned and boned, with all visible fat removed. Broil, boil, barbecue, microwave, roast or "fry" in a nonstick pan using only a cooking spray.

Whoa! Before you head off to the store to buy your food, you should know that you're better off sticking to the protein list rather than venturing into the grocery store or health-food store for "protein bars." Most of those bars contain too many carbohydrates and not enough protein. Go figure.

And while we have your attention, here's a reminder to keep your carb intake to 80 to 100 grams (see page 45 on how to read a food label).

Also, (we're nag, nag, nagging again), be sure to gulp your water and don't forget to swallow a vitamin.

YOUR SPACE

DAY FOUR

DAILY ACTION PLAN

• Day

• Date

• BREAKFAST

Healthy snack

• LUNCH

Healthy snack

• DINNER

Occasional Dessert

How Many Carbs?

How Much Fat?

Vitamins?

Yep! Nope.

How much Water?

Weight?

How Many Steps?

• For Exercise, I

• I Am Great because

• My Dream is

• To reach it, today I will

• If happens, I will

• My reward today is

O.K. So Instead I'm On www.bodypride.com

DAY FIVE

Change isn't easy. You'll find that eating differently means that sometimes you'll be inconvenienced. You'll have to carry the menu with you when you're food shopping or eating out. You'll have to read labels and consider every bite of food before you stick it in your mouth. Whine, whine, whine.

You'll survive. Trust us. After a few days, you'll know pretty much what's on the menu (sea bass, yogurt and Chinese pea pods) and what isn't (hot fudge and fried anythings). Remind yourself that your body's nipping away at extra fat, you're getting good results, you're feeling less hungry and your energy is high. And you're making changes that will benefit you for life.

"I don't see the diet as depriving me. It's not that I can't have something, but that I don't want it right now. I can eat it later, when I'm in better shape. I want to make the right food choices now."

YOUR SPACE

DAY FIVE

DAILY ACTION PLAN

• Day ....

• Date ....

• BREAKFAST ....

....

Healthy snack ....

....

• LUNCH ....

....

Healthy snack ....

....

• DINNER ....

....

Occasional Dessert ....

How Many Carbs? How Much Fat?

Vitamins? Yep! Nope.

How much Water?

Weight?

How Many Steps?

• For Exercise, I ....

....

• I Am Great because ....

....

• My Dream is ....

....

• To reach it, today I will ....

....

• If .... happens, I will ....

....

• My reward today is ....

O.K. So Instead I'm On www.bodypride.com

DAY SIX

How's it going? Has the menu brainwashed you into eating three well-balanced meals a day? Hope so, if not, adjust your thinking. If you start skipping now, you'll slow down your metabolism, that squirrel-like rate at which you burn calories. Don't lower its activity by starving it.

A survey by the National Centers for Disease Control and Prevention found high school students thought there were three ways to lose weight:

1. skipping meals
2. taking diet pills
3. throwing up after eating.

Hello! These are unhealthy and your body won't work under those conditions.

1. Unhealthy, starvation diets that deprive you of a balanced meal don't click. They can cause painful gallstones, hair loss, weakness and the runs. You'll crave, then binge and get nowhere. These yo-yo diets also put repeated stress on your bod.
2. Now let's slap around diet pills. In 1993, the Federal Drug Administration decided that 111 ingredients in diet pills didn't work or posed serious health risks. Some make the inside of your stomach swell to give you a false sense of fullness. But the chemical used to do that can cause blockage in the throat and stomach.
3. And who wants to throw up? Besides, it's just wrong. See page 82 on eating disorders to get the whole nasty list on what this does to your teeth, your health and your friendships.

On the *bodyPRIDE* diet, you'll learn about healthy foods that can carry you through life. Over the past 25 years, we've proven that it's safe and effective with thousands of teens.

YOUR SPACE

DAY SIX

DAILY ACTION PLAN

• Day ....

• Date ....

• BREAKFAST ....

....

Healthy snack ....

....

• LUNCH ....

....

Healthy snack ....

....

• DINNER ....

....

Occasional Dessert ....

How Many Carbs? How Much Fat?

Vitamins? Yep! Nope.

How much Water?

Weight?

How Many Steps?

• For Exercise, I ....

....

• I Am Great because ....

....

• My Dream is ....

....

• To reach it, today I will ....

....

• If .... happens, I will ....

....

• My reward today is ....

O.K. So Instead I'm On www.bodypride.com

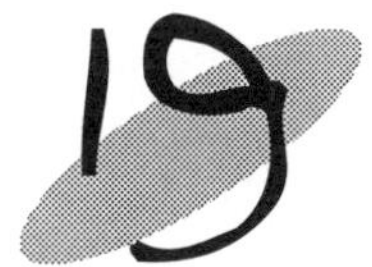

NON-BETTY CROCKERS

Things are going fine as you start the second week into your new way of eating. You're weighing yourself every day and feeling lighter, healthier, fitter. Then a nagging thought crowds into your head: why not eat something that's not on the list?

Now, of course, you'll immediately turn back to Chapter 13 and review all the nifty tricks you can play to ward off cravings and impulses. You can wait it out, knowing it's temporary. You can invest some time in gentle exercise and neck massages. You won't jeopardize being in ketosis, which reduces hunger and all those cravings. You will avoid people, places and situations that make you want to go crazy.

Yeah, yeah, yeah. You've heard it all before.

Well, there's even another way to battle those thoughts telling you to tamper with the menu: You can stay legit and still get creative.

Try something on the menu that you haven't eaten before (Puffed Kashi, anyone?). Or if you have tried it before, try it a different way. Like spinach, for instance. Ask your friends how they eat it—how about raw in a salad or steamed with white vinegar on top. Maybe frozen in a Popeye sicle?

Scattered throughout this chapter are favorite recipes from teens, beginning with:

RICK'S QUICK FIX LUNCH

"I take a 3 1/2 ounce can of white chicken, empty out the water (and now it's only 2 1/2 ounces), dump it onto a plate, throw some sugar-free barbecue sauce on it and microwave it for 60 seconds. It's hot and it's hearty."

DAY SEVEN

You've conquered cravings, but maybe your friend is having a problem with chocolate calling her, gently whispering, "I'm here, take me!" What can you tell her?

1. Don't buy it. Instead, use that money for something positive, like traveling or clothes. Remember, cravings cost you.
2. Keep your distance. Take out a restraining order against it. Don't allow it in your home, backpack or locker. Run away if it's offered to you.
3. Avoid your danger zones. Don't walk past a vending machine if you can go another way. Don't stroll down the goodie aisle in the grocery store. Don't hang out at a friend's house where the coffee table is laden down with bowls of melt-in-your-mouth globules.
4. Become independent. Whenever you feel tempted, remember that you're in control...no one else.

LUNCH ANYONE?

Dijon green beans:

Whisk together 1 tablespoon vinegar, 1 teaspoon Dijon mustard, 2 cloves minced garlic, 1/2 teaspoon oregano and 1/8 teaspoon black pepper. Pour over 1 pound steamed green beans and toss to coat. Measure out a portion and enjoy it.

SARA'S VEGGIE SPLASH

"I put tons of vegetables, asparagus, celery, cucumbers, okra, different kinds of pepper, raw spinach, tomatoes and zucchini into a juicer and knock 'em around until they're pulverized. Then I cool it in the fridge and drink it frosty, a cup at a time, to get my veg portion in. Most of the time, it tastes great. But sometimes the concoction is a little too...out there"

DAY SEVEN

DAILY ACTION PLAN

• Day ....

• Date ....

• BREAKFAST ....

....

Healthy snack ....

....

• LUNCH ....

....

Healthy snack ....

....

• DINNER ....

....

Occasional Dessert ....

How Many Carbs? How Much Fat?

Vitamins? Yep! Nope.

How much Water?

Weight?

How Many Steps?

• For Exercise, I ....

....

• I Am Great because ....

....

• My Dream is ....

....

• To reach it, today I will ....

....

• If .... happens, I will ....

....

• My reward today is ....

O.K. So Instead I'm On www.bodypride.com

DAY EIGHT

OK, here's the question you've been wanting to ask: "Can I substitute certain foods on the menu with foods that have the same number of calories?"

And we'll answer: No. You know why? Because you need to follow the menu carefully to get max nutrition and weight loss. Don't play with the chemistry. Foods that have the same number of calories may be higher in carbs than those on the menu.

Some meats and fish are not on the menu because they're too high in fat and calories (like pastrami and pork). Also, some frozen "diet" meals from the supermarket are low in protein and high in calories, carbs and fat. So much for the "diet" part of the package label.

Now, aren't you glad you asked?

The Journal of the American Dietetic Association will send you free information on its Child Nutrition & Health Campaign if you send a self-addressed, stamped envelope to: ADA-Child Nutrition Fact Sheet, 216 W. Jackson Blvd., Chicago, Illinois 60606, or call, 800-877-1600.

TAKE A CHANCE

It's the end of your first week of dieting. Take a sec to measure yourself in the same five spots you did on Prep Day 2:

- chest _______
- waist _______
- lower abdomen _______
- hips _______
- and upper thigh _______

Mark it all down here. Be patient. Inches take awhile to shrink.

BEFORE YOU CHOW DOWN

Share your creation with the world. Post your favorite recipe at our web site, **www.bodypride.com**.

YOUR SPACE

DAY EIGHT

DAILY ACTION PLAN

• Day

• Date

• BREAKFAST

Healthy snack

• LUNCH

Healthy snack

• DINNER

Occasional Dessert

How Many Carbs?

How Much Fat?

Vitamins?

Yep! Nope.

How much Water?

Weight?

How Many Steps?

• For Exercise, I

• I Am Great because

• My Dream is

• To reach it, today I will

• If happens, I will

• My reward today is

O.K. So Instead I'm On www.bodypride.com

DAY NINE

Ready for another recipe? Before you get to Darcy's, let's look at Your Recipe. If you were to write down your recipe for a healthy life, what ingredients would there be?

____

____

____

____

____

Your recipe is sure to be different from ours, but maybe not by much. We list it this kinda-corny-but real way:

H Higher purpose

E Eating healthy food

A Activity

L Laughter and play

T Time alone

H Human contact

Higher purpose: People feel good when they're doing something important. When they're committed to ideas that are bigger than themselves and give without expecting something back. What do you believe in? How often do you lend your time and talent to causes that matter to you?

Want to lend a hand by volunteering in your area? Or need a mentor to show you the ropes? Call ABC Children First One-to-One Mentoring Hotline at 800-914-2212. You'll automatically be connected to your community's volunteer center. Isn't technology great?

The Department of Education has a free student's guide on how to get involved in your community called "Catch the Spirit" and the Department of the Interior has a free brochure on "Why Save Endangered Species?" Get either or both by writing to the Consumer Information Center, Dept. 588C and 578C, Pueblo, Colorado 81009 . Or you can download the information at http://www.pueblo.gsa.gov. For more information, call 202-501-1794.

Eating healthy food: Even though you're on a special diet now, you'll want to continue to eat healthy foods forever. That means fruits and vegetables, protein for energy and muscle building, moderate carbohydrates and little fat.

Activity: Your body was designed for movement. Just look at it, all those swinging parts. (Feel free to re-read Chapter 4 for more details.)

Laughter and play: When you laugh—except during a serious part in class—you're doing yourself a favor. Your body, brain and relationships work better. Even during bad times, we can find one thing to feel good about. Go ahead, we challenge you to find it.

Time alone: When you spend time alone, you give yourself a chance to recharge. Even the Energizer Bunny has down time, off camera. Read without the radio or TV on or go for a solo walk. You'll like the thoughts that come flying into your head when you're not distracted.

Human contact: Like a puppy, if you don't get enough attention and affection from other people, you'll whimper, get depressed and sometimes even get sick. Fortunately, unlike puppies, you can link up with others (imagine a little dog doing a conference call with Spike and Spitzy down the street). How good are you at staying connected? If the calls and invites aren't coming in, you make the call.

HEALTH: It's a recipe that tastes and feels good.

DARCY'S BLACKBERRIES PILE

"I don't like fruits because they're like grandma food—dates and casaba melons, like what are those even? But I tested some blackberries, and I think the texture is really nice. And they look like alien food. So I just grab a handful, that's about 2/3 cup, like the menu says, and they're carryable. A 4-ounce glass of orange juice in the morning is also an easy way to get my fruit in."

AND FOR DINNER

Curried chicken:

Combine 1/2 cup plain nonfat yogurt with 1/2 cup fat-free mayonnaise, 4 tablespoons finely chopped onions, 1 teaspoon ginger and 1 teaspoon curry powder. Combine 1 teaspoon paprika, 1/2 teaspoon black pepper and sprinkle over chicken. Toss until coated. Spray a nonstick skillet with nonstick spray and cook chicken over a medium heat until cooked through, about 3 to 4 minutes. Stir in yogurt mixture, one tablespoon per serving. (Store the rest in the fridge for later.). Cook for 2 minutes.

DAY NINE

DAILY ACTION PLAN

• Day

• Date

• BREAKFAST

Healthy snack

• LUNCH

Healthy snack

• DINNER

Occasional Dessert

How Many Carbs? How Much Fat?

Vitamins?

Yep! Nope.

How much Water?

Weight?

How Many Steps?

• For Exercise, I

• I Am Great because

• My Dream is

• To reach it, today I will

• If happens, I will

• My reward today is

O.K. So Instead I'm On www.bodypride.com

20

ROCKIN'

It's time we talked about sweating again. As you're cruising along on the diet and writing all over your DAP, we hope we've left you enough space under the exercise section to pencil in everything you're doing. Whether it's a full-out sport or just a little movement, it's all important.

Remember that exercise improves your fat-burning capacity, revs up your metabolism, quiets cravings and jump-starts your mood by releasing "happy" endorphins throughout your system. Exercise improves your circulation, which pumps up your heart and lung function, and speeds up the delivery of blood and oxygen to your cells. This stress-reliever also gives you time with yourself. That means you can think about what's going on in your life.

But that's not all. Exercise also increases the mitochondria in your body. You remember, those trillion, tiny eggs in your cells that serve as fat-burning furnaces. The more of these in your cells, the easier it is for you to burn stored fat for fuel.

C'mon. Be a Mitochondriac(TR). Exercise.

"I work at a gym and people come in there all the time when they're like age 35 or something. They now want to do something with their bodies and they're mad that they look and feel the lousy way they do. They could of been exposed to fitness a long time ago. Look at how many years they've missed."

DAY TEN

Does your exercise routine thrill you? If not, make a change. Try something new. Buddy up with a friend. Strap on some headsets. And get this, dancing—to rap, heavy metal, classic or gothic rock, even disco, swing, you name it—counts as exercise.

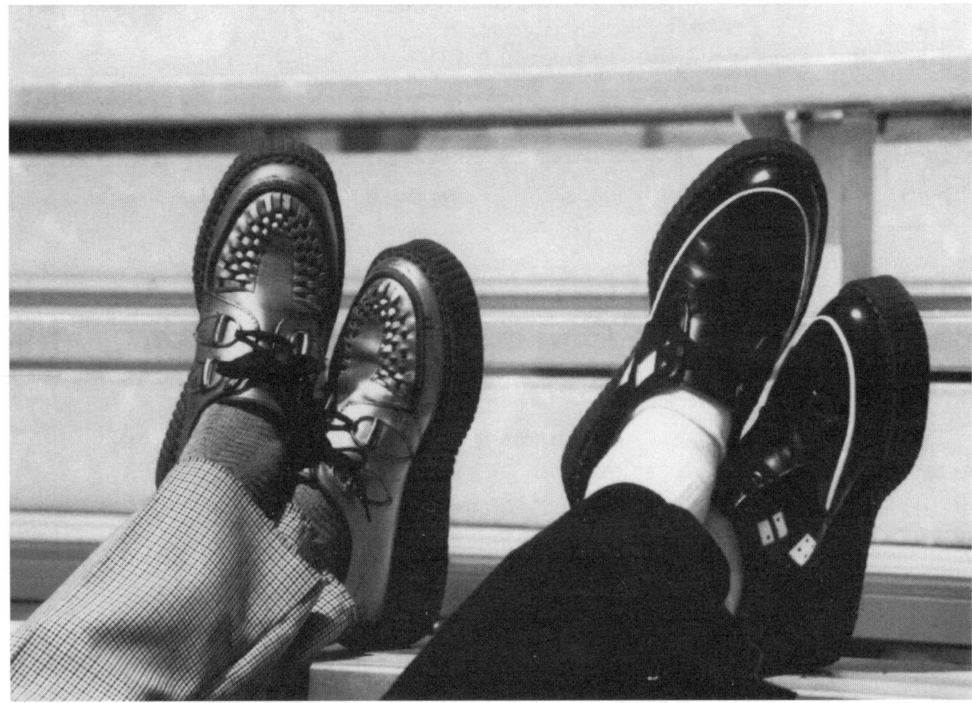

One warning: There are times when you shouldn't exert yourself. Skip your regular exercise whenever you have a fever (if it's caused by a viral infection, exercise can push the virus into your heart muscle). Also lay low after any injury or surgery. Talk to a doctor or nurse first. If you've been away from your usual routine for four or more days, ease back into it. Don't try to make up for lost time. That's when you're more likely to injure yourself.

Does this mean it's OK to skip a day if you don't feel like exercising? Uh, like nice try. When you're dragging, that's the time when you need exercise the most. Now get moving.

YOUR SPACE

DAY TEN

DAILY ACTION PLAN

• Day ....

• Date ....

• BREAKFAST ....

....

Healthy snack ....

....

• LUNCH ....

....

Healthy snack ....

....

• DINNER ....

....

Occasional Dessert ....

How Many Carbs? How Much Fat?

Vitamins? ☐ Yep! ☐ Nope.

How much Water?

Weight?

How Many Steps?

• For Exercise, I ....

....

• I Am Great because ....

....

• My Dream is ....

....

• To reach it, today I will ....

....

• If .... happens, I will ....

....

• My reward today is ....

O.K. So Instead I'm On www.bodypride.com

DAY ELEVEN

How's your DAP doing? Has it become a record of your first 10 days of improvement or have you ignored it? It's not too late to start marking it up. Remember, if you have a setback, you don't have to return to start. Just number your DAP with today's date and move onward. Next week, you'll have something good to review.

DAY ELEVEN

DAILY ACTION PLAN

• Day ....

• Date ....

• BREAKFAST ....

Healthy Snack ....

• LUNCH ....

Healthy Snack ....

• DINNER ....

Occasional Dessert ....

How Many Carbs? [ ] How Much Fat? [ ]

Vitamins? [ ] Yep! [ ] Nope.

How much Water? [ ]

Weight? [ ]

How Many Steps? [ ]

• For Exercise, I ....

• I Am Great because ....

• My Dream is ....

• To reach it, today I will ....

• If .... happens, I will ....

• My reward today is ....

O.K. So Instead I'm On www.bodypride.com

DAY TWELVE

Smart Man Talking: Dr. Marshall Stamper, who has helped people lose weight since 1971, reminds us to be good to ourselves. He says, "Most of us are more willing to forgive others than to forgive ourselves. When you make a mistake on the diet—or in life—learn from it and move on. Mistakes don't define us. How we recover from them does."

TAKE A CHANCE

Stuff That's Gross About Some People	**Stuff That's Gross About Me**
meanness	NOTHING!!!!!!!!
rudeness	
self-mutilation	
exposed butt cracks	
whiny voices	
sloppiness	
body odor	
smelly breath	
no deodorant	
public scratching	
groping in public	
dirty nails	
______________	
______________	
______________	
______________	
______________	
______________	
______________	
______________	
______________	
______________	
______________	
______________	

DAY TWELVE

DAILY ACTION PLAN

• Day

• Date

• BREAKFAST

Healthy snack

• LUNCH

Healthy snack

• DINNER

Occasional Dessert

How Many Carbs?

How Much Fat?

Vitamins?

Yep! Nope.

How much Water?

Weight?

How Many Steps?

• For Exercise, I

• I Am Great because

• My Dream is

• To reach it, today I will

• If happens, I will

• My reward today is

O.K. So Instead I'm On www.bodypride.com

21

POWER THE SYSTEM

Maybe you were just hanging out and suddenly you got an idea to do something that's a blast. You just had to make it happen. Or maybe something sad hit and you found this heat inside firing you up to fix a part of your life. You thought about it, then did what had to be done. You motivated yourself to create a plan, Your Plan.

An excellent first step. But remember you have to stay motivated, all the way. You can't stay turned on and committed one day, then lose it and become Beavis and Butt-head the next. Heh-Heh, motivation sucks.

No way. Motivation gets you where you want to be.

Kyle remembers: "In the beginning, the thing I want is all I ever think about. It's like burning a hole in my head and taking control of me. But after a few days, I get distracted and stop thinking about it. To remind myself why I was motivated in the first place, I make a list of my reasons—all the good I was going to get out of it. Then, if I start feeling unmotivated, I look at the list and get going again."

Remember your motivation cards, you know, those index cards mentioned on page 11 where you wrote down what you wanted and why. Where are they? Under the bed? Buried inside your desk? Find them. Stick 'em in your pocket, wallet or backpack. No one else has to see them but you. They're your ticket to getting to a better place.

"I kinda think of my goal as my job, my other job, other than school. I tell myself that my reward, the reason I'm doing this, is like a paycheck. A big paycheck."

DAY THIRTEEN

Got the motivation blahs? Decide what's causing them. Have you figured out what you want? Have you made some progress toward getting it? Have you stopped long enough to congratulate yourself when you've made progress? Maybe someone can help encourage you. Who can you call now who can help get you back in the groove?

DAY THIRTEEN

DAILY ACTION PLAN

• Day

• Date

• BREAKFAST

Healthy snack

• LUNCH

Healthy snack

• DINNER

Occasional Dessert

How Many Carbs?

How Much Fat?

Vitamins?

Yep! Nope.

How much Water?

Weight?

How Many Steps?

• For Exercise, I

• I Am Great because

• My Dream is

• To reach it, today I will

• If happens, I will

• My reward today is

O.K. So Instead I'm On www.bodypride.com

DAY FOURTEEN

Here's a rhyme for you:

The more enthused,
the more you lose.

You don't have to be a poetry scholar to figure out this one: The higher your interest and enthusiasm the more you'll succeed. The hard part is keeping your motivation from disappearing into a black hole. "Bite the nail" and stick with it.

"I learned many good lessons from my years ice skating. I learned that one mistake will not kill you. I won a competition even though I fell out of a jump and received a slight deduction. You have to pull yourself together and forget about what you did before. You're on to something else now."

TAKE A CHANCE

People in the military wear dog tags that identify them. Usually, it's their name, rank and serial number. Imagine you have 36 letters that would describe who you are on a military dog tag. What words would you use? Who are you and who do you want to be?

☐	☐	☐	☐	☐	☐	☐	☐	☐	☐	☐	☐
☐	☐	☐	☐	☐	☐	☐	☐	☐	☐	☐	☐
☐	☐	☐	☐	☐	☐	☐	☐	☐	☐	☐	☐

"My dog tag says, 'Joey, The Chick Magnet of Jersey.' "

You can actually get one of these dog tags. The Smithsonian Air & Space Museum in Washington, DC. can customize one for you. So can local pet stores. Really.

DAY FOURTEEN

DAILY ACTION PLAN

• Day

• Date

• BREAKFAST

Healthy snack

• LUNCH

Healthy snack

• DINNER

Occasional Dessert

How Many Carbs?

How Much Fat?

Vitamins?

Yep! Nope.

How much Water?

Weight?

How Many Steps?

• For Exercise, I

• I Am Great because

• My Dream is

• To reach it, today I will

• If ______ happens, I will

• My reward today is

O.K. So Instead I'm On www.bodypride.com

DAY FIFTEEN

Here's a big secret: it's not always true that the most talented or even the luckiest person wins. You've seen this happen before. The smartest kid in the class bombs a test. The strongest athlete chokes in the last seconds of the game. While others get sidetracked or distracted, the teen who finishes proudly is the one who stays focused. You're about halfway through this program. Can you count on you to make it?

"If I didn't have the passion for theater, the drive, the fire, I wouldn't have lasted this long, considering all the shows I've tried out for and been rejected. I'm proud of the persistence and the self-esteem that I've taken from my experience."

BEFORE YOU HEAD OUT THE DOOR

Find that tape measure and get an up-to-date reading of your:

- chest _______
- waist _______
- lower abdomen _______
- hips _______
- and upper thigh _______

YOUR SPACE

DAY FIFTEEN

DAILY ACTION PLAN

• Day ....

• Date ....

• BREAKFAST ....

....

Healthy snack ....

....

• LUNCH ....

....

Healthy snack ....

....

• DINNER ....

....

Occasional Dessert ....

How Many Carbs? [ ] How Much Fat? [ ]

Vitamins? [ ] Yep! [ ] Nope.

How much Water? [ ]

Weight? [ ]

How Many Steps? [ ]

• For Exercise, I ....

....

• I Am Great because ....

....

• My Dream is ....

....

• To reach it, today I will ....

....

• If .... happens, I will ....

....

• My reward today is ....

O.K. So Instead I'm On www.bodypride.com

22

TOO FULL OR TOO EMPTY

Vinnie didn't get invited to the party. While he's pacing around the kitchen, he reaches for a bag of chips. Lonely, depressed, empty, food.

Linda left her uniform for the big game in her mother's car. The coach won't let her play without it. She sits in the bleachers, scarfing cookies. She wants to kill him. Stress, anxiety, food.

Vinnie and Linda use food to cover feelings of depression, powerlessness and anxiety.

They are not alone. In our culture, food is more than a source of fuel. It's comfort, companionship, reward, punishment, escape, control and power. As babies, bottles are shoved into our mouths to quiet us. As kids, we're rewarded for good behavior with cookies and candy. How many times was dessert the payoff for cleaning our plates, even when it meant gobbling more than we wanted or needed? Then there were the threats of no goodies at all when we were bad.

Think about it: Eat your spinach and you can have cake. Win the game and we'll all go out for pizza. You've heard these, so it's no wonder we think about and use food to deal with stress and to reward ourselves for good deeds.

As you read in Chapter 15, there are better ways to handle stress and anxiety. Remember exercise? Remember giving yourself enough time? Remember identifying stressers and figuring out ways to manage them? And remember the final thought: Food rewards are for babies. Got it? Good.

DAY SIXTEEN

Just as stress leads to anxiety, feelings of loneliness and emptiness can make you feel empty and depressed. Using food at times like these will only make you feel worse. Don't cover your feelings with food. Get active. Do something you'll be able to feel good about later. Take a walk, write a letter, blast your favorite song, give a bag of fruit to a homeless shelter.

Take charge. Complete this sentence: I'm unhappy when ______________

____

This is what I can do about it to feel better: ______________

____

DAY SIXTEEN

DAILY ACTION PLAN

• Day

• Date

• BREAKFAST

Healthy snack

• LUNCH

Healthy snack

• DINNER

Occasional Dessert

How Many Carbs?

How Much Fat?

Vitamins?

Yep! Nope.

How much Water?

Weight?

How Many Steps?

• For Exercise, I

• I Am Great because

• My Dream is

• To reach it, today I will

• If happens, I will

• My reward today is

O.K. So Instead I'm On www.bodypride.com

DAY SEVENTEEN

Uh-oh, you just hit a wall. You're zipping along, following the menu and being active, but you're not dropping pounds. Your bathroom scale is just stuck on some stupid number and it won't move, no matter how much you yell at it.

Cool down, it happens. It even has a name: a plateau. Yeah, it's kind of a French word meaning things have stalled, evened out or topped off. Even though you're following the program, your body is resisting change. And you're thinking, this isn't fair. Why the punishment?

First, look at your little pal, the ketostick. If it's not a shade of purple, ask yourself if carbs have slipped into your food somehow—like aliens dripped some high-carb marinade on your chicken. Or carbs were hiding out in your hot chocolate mix. It's time to be a detective and locate those hidden meanies before they do major damage and stall your progress.

Are you measuring carefully? Eating ALL the foods? If you skip the fruit at lunch that doesn't mean you can have a super big salad with dinner. Remember, there's a chemistry to all of this.

If you're in ketosis, the stalled scale might be because your body's holding onto water. Add lemon to your water and it should even things out again (but don't give up drinking water—that will set you way back).

You can break past a plateau. Here's how: Don't lose your momentum. Look over your DAP and make sure you're not cutting corners.

You may need to switch to this Plateau Menu until you lose 1½ pounds. But don't use it for more than three days. (And don't use the Plateau Menu when you're not facing a plateau, otherwise it won't work when you really need it.) Did you get all that? OK, now the menu:

PLATEAU MENU

Breakfast

1 egg or egg substitute (boiled, poached or cooked with nonstick spray in a nonstick pan)
1/2 grapefruit or 4 ounces of grapefruit juice
Choice of any calorie-free beverage

Lunch

3-1/2 ounces of white fish
1/2 cup of cooked spinach
1/2 grapefruit or 4 ounces of grapefruit juice
1 cup of lettuce
Choice of any calorie-free beverage

Dinner

3-1/2 ounces of white fish
1/2 cup of cooked spinach
1/2 grapefruit or 4 ounces of grapefruit juice
1 cup of lettuce
Choice of any calorie-free beverage

At Bedtime

1 cup of hot lemon water (boil 1/4 of a lemon in water for three minutes or microwave it for 1-1/2 minutes).

DAY SEVENTEEN

DAILY ACTION PLAN

• Day

• Date

• BREAKFAST

Healthy snack

• LUNCH

Healthy snack

• DINNER

Occasional Dessert

How Many Carbs?

How Much Fat?

VITAMINS?

Yep! Nope.

How much WATER?

WEIGHT?

How MANY STEPS?

• For Exercise, I

• I Am Great because

• My Dream is

• To reach it, today I will

• If happens, I will

• My reward today is

O.K. So Instead I'm On www.bodypride.com

DAY EIGHTEEN

If you had to put your feelings in the washing machine, what cycle would you set them on? Cold, warm, hot, delicate, normal, heavy duty, can take a tumble and bounce back?

The message: Take care of your feelings as carefully as you would your favorite clothes.

DAY EIGHTEEN

DAILY ACTION PLAN

• Day ....

• Date ....

• BREAKFAST ....

Healthy snack ....

• LUNCH ....

Healthy snack ....

• DINNER ....

Occasional Dessert ....

How Many Carbs? How Much Fat?

Vitamins? ☐ Yep! ☐ Nope.

How much Water?

Weight?

How Many Steps?

• For Exercise, I ....

• I Am Great because ....

• My Dream is ....

• To reach it, today I will ....

• If .... happens, I will ....

• My reward today is ....

O.K. So Instead I'm On www.bodypride.com

23

LET'S BE HONEST

Over the past few weeks, there have been times when you wanted to give up. Or let a craving get the best of you. Or test the diet to see if you could eat something outside the menu and still keep burning stored fat. There's no problem admitting that.

It's pretty human. But look at the facts: you didn't drop out and if you blipped a few times, you got right back in sync. Great. You've just shown that you always have a choice as to how you react, no matter what the obstacle. You can feel bad and quit, or you can learn and grow from it.

DAY NINETEEN

We don't want to freak you out, but watching TV can make you fat. Peg Bundy never cooked a thing in her life, but even "Married...With Children" can help you put on the pounds. It's like this: Have you ever grabbed the cookies or chips as you flipped to your favorite show, only to realize half an hour later that the bag was empty?

When your attention is focused somewhere else, like on that star of "Baywatch" or "Melrose Place," you aren't thinking about what and how much you're shoveling in your mouth.

It's easy to stop this:

1. Just make a point of eating in one place in your house, like the kitchen or at the dining room table.
2. When you're eating, think about your food.
3. Turn off the TV, put aside other distractions and simply enjoy the taste, texture and smell of the chow.

YOUR SPACE

DAY NINETEEN

DAILY ACTION PLAN

• Day ....

• Date ....

• BREAKFAST ....

....

Healthy snack ....

....

• LUNCH ....

....

Healthy snack ....

....

• DINNER ....

....

Occasional Dessert ....

How Many Carbs? [ ] How Much Fat? [ ]

Vitamins? [ ] Yep! [ ] Nope.

How much Water? [ ]

Weight? [ ]

How Many Steps? [ ]

• For Exercise, I ....

....

• I Am Great because ....

....

• My Dream is ....

....

• To reach it, today I will ....

....

• If .... happens, I will ....

....

• My reward today is ....

O.K. So Instead I'm On www.bodypride.com

DAY TWENTY

Brian knows this about scaling the heights: "Weighing myself every day doesn't mean that I'm obsessing about how much I weigh. My friend doesn't get on the scale too often, and that works for her. But I think if I didn't keep things in check, over time I would get carried away and gain weight. Now I get on the scale and I reassure myself that I'm eating right and exercising."

Weigh yourself the same way and time every day. The best way is naked, the best time is first thing in the morning after you've gone to the bathroom.

Enough said.

WHAT STUFF WEIGHS

- Nike tennis shoes: 2-1/2 pounds
- Dr. Martens: 8 pounds
- 501s: 3 pounds
- a six-pack of soda: 72 ounces
- a chain wallet, empty: 2 ounces
- hair extensions: 4 ounces
- 10 acrylic nails: 1 ounce
- your breath: 0 ounces
- a skateboard: 5 pounds
- a pager: 6 ounces
- a phone number on a Post-it note: 0 ounces
- a bikini top: 2 ounces
- a thong bottom: 2 ounces
- board shorts, wet and sandy: 3 pounds
- Oakley sunglasses: 3 ounces
- boxers: 4 ounces
- briefs: 4 ounces

DAY TWENTY

DAILY ACTION PLAN

- Day
- Date

- BREAKFAST

Healthy snack

- LUNCH

Healthy snack

- DINNER

Occasional Dessert

How Many Carbs? How Much Fat?

Vitamins?
Yep! Nope.

How much Water?

Weight?

How Many Steps?

- For Exercise, I
- I Am Great because
- My Dream is
- To reach it, today I will
- If happens, I will
- My reward today is

O.K. So Instead I'm On www.bodypride.com

DAY TWENTY-ONE

"I lost some weight and everyone kept saying that I looked thinner in the face. Hey, maybe that's the first thing they notice, but what about the rest of me? Check it out!"

Are you waiting for piles of praise to fall your way? Well, how are you at rewarding yourself? Maybe you could divide up the weight you have to lose into five parts and give yourself a present for each time you reach 1/5th of your goal. A concert ticket? CD? Short trip? Movie? Sheet music? Clothes? Magazines? Time to do nothing?

TAKE A CHANCE

The speed dial on a phone makes connecting faster and easier than the old-fashioned way of pushing all those digits, one by one. If you could speed dial 10 things that make you happy, what would they be and why? Talking to your best friend? Going to the mall? Helping someone out? Perfecting a move on your skateboard, bike or Rollerblades?

1. __________
2. __________
3. __________
4. __________
5. __________
6. __________
7. __________
8. __________
9. __________
10. __________

DAY TWENTY-ONE

DAILY ACTION PLAN

• Day

• Date

• BREAKFAST

Healthy snack

• LUNCH

Healthy snack

• DINNER

Occasional Dessert

How Many Carbs?

How Much Fat?

Vitamins?

Yep!

Nope.

How much Water?

Weight?

How Many Steps?

• For Exercise, I

• I Am Great because

• My Dream is

• To reach it, today I will

• If happens, I will

• My reward today is

O.K. So Instead I'm On www.bodypride.com

HELP IS HERE

Jeff is ashamed of his family. His parents are loud and always fighting. His brothers and sisters are bratty and mess with Jeff's stuff. And the house is a disaster, crammed with junk inside and out. No one wants to clean it up.

Jeff is 14 and stays clear of his home as much as he can, hanging out at the fast-food joint on the corner or the movie theater, eating junk food and wishing he lived some place else...with other people. When he has to be home, he stays in his room, in front of the TV, trying to ignore the noise and bad feelings. He also eats, all the time, and thinks how things will be different if he ever has kids.

Is there anything Jeff can do now to climb out of this?

WHAT WOULD YOU SAY?

Solving a problem starts with doing something really obvious: State the problem. What's going on with Jeff?

____

____

____

____

____

You might have written something like, "Jeff isn't happy with his family and he stays away from home and eats too much junk food."

The second step to solving a problem is to create a list of possible solutions. Don't worry if they'll all work for Jeff or not, just write them down. Go wild with sharp ideas.

1. ______________________________________
2. ______________________________________
3. ______________________________________
4. ______________________________________

Now, which is the best solution? Think it through, then circle the one that makes the most sense. There may be more than one solution, but circle your favorite.

The next step to solving a problem, as you learned in Chapter 2, is to create a plan. Jeff needs a goal that is big enough to matter, but small enough to achieve. For example, Jeff can start by telling his parents how he feels. Then he can ask his family and friends for help. He can also begin with himself by eating only healthy foods three times a day. He can walk or exercise to give himself time to think, instead of hiding out inside. And he can clean up his own room. By doing all of this, Jeff can set an example for his brothers and sisters and feel better about himself.

What did you come up with?

DAY TWENTY-TWO

What about you? Do you have a problem you need help solving? Do the same thing you did for Jeff:

State the problem.

____

Create a list of possible solutions.

1. ____
2. ____
3. ____
4. ____

Circle the best solution.

Set a goal.

Follow through. And while you're at it, give us a chance to praise you. We're looking for stories of how you or your friend made a plan to solve a problem and then saw it to the end. Don't be modest! E-mail us at CGraff@bodypride.com. Let us celebrate with you.

SPEAKING OF FOLLOWING THROUGH

Tape measure time. You know what to do.

- chest _______
- waist _______
- lower abdomen _______
- hips _______
- and upper thigh _______

DAY TWENTY-TWO

DAILY ACTION PLAN

• Day

• Date

• BREAKFAST

Healthy snack

• LUNCH

Healthy snack

• DINNER

Occasional Dessert

How Many Carbs?

How Much Fat?

Vitamins?

Yep! Nope.

How much Water?

Weight?

How Many Steps?

• For Exercise, I

• I Am Great because

• My Dream is

• To reach it, today I will

• If happens, I will

• My reward today is

O.K. So Instead I'm On www.bodypride.com

DAY TWENTY-THREE

You can express your dreams through words or pictures. Which do you prefer? Think of it this way: If you wanted to send a postcard to a friend about the place you're in right now, would you rather draw the front side of the postcard or write on the back? Go ahead. Find space somewhere here, in your book.

DAY TWENTY-THREE

DAILY ACTION PLAN

• Day ....

• Date ....

• BREAKFAST ....

Healthy snack ....

• LUNCH ....

Healthy snack ....

• DINNER ....

Occasional Dessert ....

How Many Carbs? How Much Fat?

Vitamins? ☐ Yep! ☐ Nope.

How much Water?

Weight?

How Many Steps?

• For Exercise, I ....

• I Am Great because ....

• My Dream is ....

• To reach it, today I will ....

• If .... happens, I will ....

• My reward today is ....

O.K. So Instead I'm On www.bodypride.com

DAY TWENTY-FOUR

There's only one important mealtime manner, and we're not talking about elbows on the table or food fights: Dinner tables should be your family's sanctuary where connection is passed along with the carrots. It's a place to start and continue simple family rituals, the actions that make your family special and unique.

Are you saying you're too busy to sit down for dinner with your family? Or it's too complicated to get everyone together at one time? Too, too, too ... much.
Eating with your family—at a table with the TV turned off—offers a plateful of benefits:

- **It's** a chance to talk about that funny thing that happened at school, a test, an athletic event, Mom's struggle with her computer, Dad's never-ending projects, whatever.
- **It's** a chance to brag about all you've accomplished. All right!
- **It's** a time for you to teach your family about proper nutrition. Bonus benefit: Eating at regular times regulates appetites and discourages snacking and overeating.
- **It's** a place to teach your younger bro and sis manners and show them how real people eat spaghetti (not through their noses).

Need more ammo to sell your family on having dinner too-gether? A Readers Digest study found that students who eat at least four meals a week with their families scored higher on academic tests and have higher self-esteem than those who don't.

You know this is true: If dinnertime is enjoyable, everyone will find a way to work it into the schedule.

HOW TO MAKE A HAPPY MEAL

First, relax. We're not talking McDonald's and little prizes here. What we're talking about is a dinner table that isn't seen as a place to be disciplined for messing up or for viewing food as punishment or reward. It's a time to laugh, get updated on family matters, spill milk...(tell the little one that the last one's optional).

To avoid the occasional "I don't like [blank]," some families prepare five healthy items and everyone chooses their favorite three. Or every family member has a night when he or she decides what's for dinner.

Other ways to add spice to dinner: Some families buy flowers once a week to zip up the look of the dinner table. Others have fun with utensils: one night, it's forks; one night, it's chopsticks; one night, it's hands.

What do you guys do? Let us know. Post your idea on the *bodyPRIDE* Web site (you know, **www.bodypride.com**).

DAY TWENTY-FOUR

DAILY ACTION PLAN

- Day ....
- Date ....

- BREAKFAST ....

  Healthy snack ....
- LUNCH ....

  Healthy snack ....
- DINNER ....

  Occasional Dessert ....

How Many Carbs? | How Much Fat?

Vitamins? ☐ Yep! ☐ Nope.

How much Water?

Weight?

How Many Steps?

- For Exercise, I ....
- I Am Great because ....
- My Dream is ....
- To reach it, today I will ....
- If .... happens, I will ....
- My reward today is ....

O.K. So Instead I'm On www.bodypride.com

25

LIFE LINES

Drip. Drip. Drip. Drop by drop, water can create a river or a canyon over time. It's the day-by-day stuff that adds up to become something major.

Just like in your life.

We asked some teens to pretend they were addressing their graduating class. Yep, they're standing on the stage with every ear turned their way. What words of wisdom would they give?

"Stay in school. Study hard. Be yourself. Accept yourself for who you are. Don't mess up your life. Take a long time to figure out who you are. Be open to life."

All good stuff to pack on your journey.

DAY TWENTY-FIVE

There's no one right time to exercise. It depends on when you like doing it (jogging in the morning makes Lulu loopy, but in the afternoon, her body's wide awake and she's raring to run). Also, consider when it's safe. Pre-dawn or after-dark jogs or walks outside can be dangerous.

Also think about the sunshine. Will high-noon rays wear you out? What about sunburn? Dehydration? Maybe early morning or late afternoon is best.

If you can't block out 20 minutes three times a week for in-your-face workouts, break the time down into mini workouts throughout the day. Recent studies show brief exertions add up to the full benefits of a longer session.

And while you're at it, pencil in some time for fun.

DAY TWENTY-FIVE

DAILY ACTION PLAN

• Day ....

• Date ....

• BREAKFAST ....

Healthy snack ....

• LUNCH ....

Healthy snack ....

• DINNER ....

Occasional Dessert ....

How Many Carbs? [ ] How Much Fat? [ ]

Vitamins? [ ] Yep! [ ] Nope.

How much Water? [ ]

Weight? [ ]

How Many Steps? [ ]

• For Exercise, I ....

• I Am Great because ....

• My Dream is ....

• To reach it, today I will ....

• If .... happens, I will ....

• My reward today is ....

O.K. So Instead I'm On www.bodypride.com

DAY TWENTY-SIX

What about the things that shouldn't stay with you? What do you leave behind? How about adding to our Junk It list?

JUNK IT!

skipping meals • skipping school • stupid sex • drugs • alcohol • doing less than you can • hanging out with losers • misplacing your trust • self-loathing • self-destruction • self-mutilation • violence • cruelty • helmet-less biking, skating, Rollerblading • unnecessary stress • egotism • racism • sexism • most other -isms • letting others get you down • negativity • keeping your feelings bottled inside • disrespect • lying • stealing • manipulating • spreading rumors • gambling/wasting money • unsafe, obnoxious driving • selling out • laziness •

______________________ (Your space)

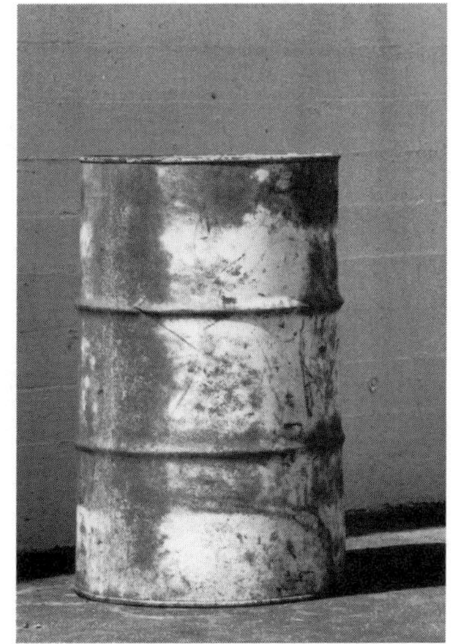

Now's a good time to check in with yourself. Are you working toward becoming the person you want to be? Look at the list and see if there's anything you need to dump. Be honest. Facing yourself is the best way to start changing things. How can you act differently? And will that benefit you?

DAY TWENTY-SIX

DAILY ACTION PLAN

- Day
- Date

- BREAKFAST

  Healthy snack

- LUNCH

  Healthy snack

- DINNER

  Occasional Dessert

How Many Carbs? How Much Fat?

Vitamins? Yep! Nope.

How much Water?

Weight?

How Many Steps?

- For Exercise, I
- I Am Great because
- My Dream is
- To reach it, today I will
- If happens, I will
- My reward today is

O.K. So Instead I'm On www.bodypride.com

DAY TWENTY-SEVEN

If you listen to some coaches, you might hear that you're too chubby for gymnastics or you're too scrawny for football. What gives?

"Football tryouts are in eight weeks, so I want to be ready for it. I've wanted to play since 5th grade but for a few years I lost interest."

When you play football, you look at the pros and figure you need to be huge. And that's true. You need padding. But muscles will move you down the field faster than fat. What's recommended is 4.6% fat-free mass to 1% body fat. A body-fat test at a gym or health clinic can clue you into your ratio. The Department of Health says the "allowable" body fat for guys age 17 to 20 is 20% and for girls is 28%.

There's an art to adding muscles without getting fat. Some body builders weigh 200 pounds but only have 10% body fat. That's pretty extreme. Some cheat and resort to steroids or other illegal drugs to attain it (need a refresher course on these guys? See Chapter 14). But it's possible to eat and exercise right to put on muscle and not fat.

Avoid really fatty foods, simple carbs and sugars—yeah, typical junk food. Eat fruits, salads as well as lean meats and other protein-rich foods (think beans, yogurt and lowfat cheese). Spend time in the gym or exercising to build a greater proportion of lean muscle mass. Do it right and you'll have no complaints.

There are plenty of people who can help you work out the right way: a coach, phys ed teacher or the buff guy pumping iron right next to you in the gym.

"The best advice my coach ever gave me was: Learn the rules. obey the rules. And no one can stop you."

DAY TWENTY-SEVEN

DAILY ACTION PLAN

• Day

• Date

• BREAKFAST

Healthy snack

• LUNCH

Healthy snack

• DINNER

Occasional Dessert

How Many Carbs?

How Much Fat?

Vitamins?

Yep! Nope.

How much Water?

Weight?

How Many Steps?

• For Exercise, I

• I Am Great because

• My Dream is

• To reach it, today I will

• If happens, I will

• My reward today is

O.K. So Instead I'm On www.bodypride.com

26

FINAL DIET DAY

Hey, look how far you've come (drum roll, please). In 28 days, you've improved your exercise output and learned how to create a lifelong plan for a safe, healthy, more enjoyable life. Don't you feel better than you did just four weeks ago?

Whatever benefits and praise have come your way are heightened by this one fact: you made it happen. You're the star here. You did it. Take a bow.

DAY TWENTY-EIGHT

Maybe today, on your last day of the diet—before you start firing up your calorie-burning metabolism—is a good day to think about all you've accomplished. Twenty-eight days is not a long time. When you were 28-days old, you just lolled around like a chubby love toy. Almost all you were good for was dribbling and thrilling your parents who couldn't stop tickling you. But look at these 28 days. You became more of the person you want to be. You did it.

You:

- **created** a plan.
- **discovered** new strategies and ideas for improving your health.
- **became** more savvy about what you do and what you should do.
- **sucked** up tons of info.
- **took** greater responsibility for your body and life.
- **faced** challenging times...and pushed through.
- **felt** *bodyPRIDE.*

TAKE A CHANCE

Think about the most important things you want to remember about:

- **Losing** fat: ________________________________
- **Exercise**: ________________________________
- **Attitude**: ________________________________

- **Taking** care of yourself: ____________________
- **The** rewards that come with all of the above: ____________________

____

____

____

____

AND JUST TO WRAP IT UP

Pull out that tape measure again and measure your:

- chest _______
- waist _______
- lower abdomen _______
- hips _______
- and upper thigh _______

What is the change from Prep Day 2?

YOUR SPACE

DAY TWENTY-EIGHT

DAILY ACTION PLAN

- Day
- Date

- BREAKFAST

  Healthy snack

- LUNCH

  Healthy snack

- DINNER

  Occasional Dessert

How Many Carbs? How Much Fat?

Vitamins?

Yep! Nope.

How much Water?

Weight?

How Many Steps?

- For Exercise, I
- I Am Great because
- My Dream is
- To reach it, today I will
- If happens, I will
- My reward today is

O.K. So Instead I'm On www.bodypride.com

27

CRANK IT UP

No one wants to be on a diet forever. Imagine it. Your friends lumbering off for pizza while you chew on that nineteenth carrot stick. Well, forget it. We're not into deprivation here.

You need a break after four weeks of eating fewer calories than you were used to eating. Your body needs a break. We're not here to torture or starve you. You'll soon be able to eat many of those foods you've been doing without. But moderation is the key.

Whether or not you reached your goal weight during the last 28 days, it's now time to learn how to make sure you don't pack it back on again. If you haven't reached your goal weight, you can return to the diet menu after you've given your body a break.

This two-week phase is called metabolic adjustment. Don't let your eyes bug out over those "Jeopardy"-sized words; the two just mean changing the rate you burn calories.

You've got to remember that we humans are just a few hundred generations away from cave people whose number one priority was survival. Your very human body is conditioned to store fuel if it feels you're losing weight. It fears that maybe, one day, no more fuel will come its way. So everything slows down to preserve what's already there. Your metabolism is calling the shots. It's time to rev it up.

You can do that by alerting your metabolism that more food is on the way and there's no reason to harbor every morsel. You do that by eating more food over a 14-day period. You'll double all your portions and since you won't be in ketosis you can eat carbs again. Hello, bread (one slice a day, please).

SORTING IT OUT

First, write here how much you weigh ____________. You won't lose any weight during this phase, but you shouldn't gain any either. If you add 1-1/2 pounds at any point, you're either eating too much or you're eating foods that aren't on the menu. Resist the urge to eat what's not on the menu.

If you happen to add a pesky 1-1/2 pounds, cut back to the weight-loss menu's portions for that day and you should be fine to move on the next day, doubling your portions and eating a slice of bread.

Also, remember the chorus: Eat three meals a day, drink water, exercise your socks off, take your vitamins, mark up your DAP and be patient. This phase only takes two weeks.

AND THEN?

After 14 days, if you haven't lost all the weight that's healthy, repeat Days 1 through 28. We don't know how many times you may need to do that—we broke our crystal ball a long time ago. It all depends on you and how much is safe to lose. Recheck the Body Mass Index chart on page 99. You may have already reached your goal weight. Remember, go for the highest number in the weight range—you've got to have something to grow into. You may also want to check in with your family doctor for guidance on what weight is right for you.

Once you've reached your goal weight, you'll enter the next and final stage, Lifetime Maintenance. It's just around the corner.

BUT FIRST

You should continue to measure yourself every week until you're happily satisfied with your progress. Measure your:

- height _______
- chest _______
- waist _______
- lower abdomen _______
- hips _______
- and upper thigh _______

YOUR SPACE

MAKE 13 MORE COPIES OF THIS!

DAILY ACTION PLAN

• Day ....

• Date ....

• BREAKFAST ....

Healthy snack ....

• LUNCH ....

Healthy snack ....

• DINNER ....

Occasional Dessert ....

How Many Carbs? How Much Fat?

Vitamins? Yep! Nope.

How much Water?

Weight?

How Many Steps?

• For Exercise, I ....

• I Am Great because ....

• My Dream is ....

• To reach it, today I will ....

• If .... happens, I will ....

• My reward today is ....

O.K. So Instead I'm On www.bodypride.com

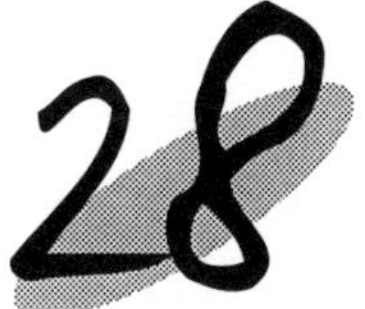

SET FOR LIFE

You've made it to your goal weight. Life is good. You may have also reached other goals along the way because you know the formula:

1. set a plan
2. stick to it
3. chart your progress every day
4. celebrate your accomplishments

There's no limit to what you can do.

Bonus: Now you're into healthy eating and exercise—good habits that will last. You really are building a better body.

But do you know that most people who lose weight don't keep it off? Ask your parents about their diet experiences and you'll probably hear some sad stories. Or just watch the news. One guy made headlines when he lost 500 pounds and became a diet spokesman for a company. But soon after he jumped back up to 700 pounds. They needed a whale platform and a gurney just to get him out of his bedroom.

That's not happening to you. You're set, because you're young and you're solid about exercise, watching your fat intake and keeping your bathroom scale nearby. If you go up or down three pounds, you won't worry about it because you know that's just a game your body plays occasionally called "hold your water" (sort of a weird version of hold your breath).

But you also know that if you go up four or more pounds and haven't grown vertically as well, you'll need to take care of business immediately. You'll stock up on proteins, veggies and fruits and cool it with the carbs, sugars and heavy fats until you're back to a healthy weight. (You may want to review the easy ways to cut back on page 44.)

"I still eat at McDonald's and eat chocolate every once in a while but I balance my food. I'll go, 'I haven't had fries or a hamburger in a while, so why not?' "

It's only natural that we would want to test our body to see how far we can push it. We may scarf some double cheese, triple pepperoni pizza one day and not gain an ounce (though this is unlikely since the salt in the pizza sauce and pepperoni and olives may do a sponge act and absorb so much water in your body that you'll be feeling like an aquarium's inside you). But let's just say, you pigout and don't gain weight.

Once.

So you're thinking, "Let's do that again."

So you do it again a few days later and you still stay the same weight.

So now you're thinking that your weight has stabilized and you'll never have to consider how or what you eat ever again. Isn't that a nice dream? Some teens are lucky and this dream comes true. But for most of us, overeating and under-exercising means our bell-bottoms will be more belled at the top than at the bottom.

If you find that you've licked up the Hefty Platter too many times, Relax. A few pounds gained isn't worthy of full-out panic mode. But recognize that you're building a pattern and if you continue to add one, two or three pounds without adding height, within a few months or years, that extra weight will mount up and be harder to knock off.

Don't let that happen. You've worked too hard to lose control of the steering wheel. You should be able to eat everything you want in healthy portions, even the occasional dunking into the fat vat. You know how your body reacts to food—revved up or slowed to a crawl. And so eating food shouldn't be a problem—or a goal—for you. You got it that food is only fuel.

Choice is the word here. It's a daily decision to care for yourself.

"When my friends and I go out, we're out late and the only places to eat are fast-food places. I order a salad and bring my own little package of fat-free dressing."

BEFORE YOU POP THAT SODA CAN

Maintaining your weight may have as much to do with what you drink as what you eat, says a report by the New York Hospital-Cornell Medical Center:

Fact: The average teenager drinks 64.5 gallons of soft drinks a year, which is three times as much as your parents drank in high school.

Fact: Drinking the wrong stuff can cause bone fractures (due to deficient calcium intake), tooth decay and tooth tissue damage (due to excess sugar), dehydration (due to diuretic drinks that force you to go to the bathroom all the time), and extra, sneaky pounds from high-calorie, no-nutrition drinks.

OK, don't wig out. Your throat doesn't have to become a dust pit.

Try these ideas:

- **Mix** sparkling mineral water into your high-calorie fruit drinks. You'll reduce the calories and make it easier to digest.
- **Eat** water-abundant fruits: watermelon, grapes, cantaloupe...

◆ **Keep** a cold glass of water in the fridge so you reach for that instead of a chillin' aluminum can of something else.

For a free copy of the teens-are-downing-too-much-soda report, write to Liquid Intake and Childhood Obesity, New York-Cornell Nutrition Information Center, 515 E. 71st Street, New York, NY 10021 or call 212-746-1617.

portionSENSE

The words "portion control" may sound like something the fat cops do with batons and tickets. But the size of what you eat is something everyone needs to patrol...for life. As a nation, we're all eating 300 more calories a day than we did just 10 years ago. That's because the size of our food is growing (a strange, but interesting idea for a horror movie: "The Muffin That Ate Manhattan").

No joke.

The American Dietetic Association says muffins should be 1-1/2 ounces but some cafes sell them 10-times that size. A small hamburger patty is about 1-1/2 ounces, yet we cram 12 ouncers—almost the size of baseball mitts—into our faces. Cookies, too, have grown out of control. The ADA says two ChipsAhoy!-size cookies are cool, but how many times have we downed one that's the size of a small Frisbee?

Don't think we're just bashing fat food. You can also eat too much of the "right" food. Do salads the size of the corn field in "Field of Dreams" seem skimpy to you? Well, it's time to take control.

If the words "portion control" chill you, look at it this way instead: think of it as "portionSENSE." Either way, the word "control" shouldn't conjure bad images—as long as you're the one in control. Better you control your food—or work or play—than it controlling you.

So, how can you make portionSENSE? Consider the size of a typical plate of airplane food. That's the right amount of food per meal that a person needing 2,000 calories a day should eat. Most of us fall into this category.

Sure, it may seem like little, teeny portions at first glance. That's because we're used to eating so much more. Take restaurants for example. A typical restaurant portion is the amount of food a very active, 5'10" man needs to eat at each meal to maintain his weight. That may be too much food for you.

Restaurants love stuffing you out because they think that makes you happy. As they say in the hash-slinging biz, no one comes to a restaurant to lose weight. Pizza Hut pushes its 21-slices in its Bigfoot Pizza, perfect for the mythical half man/half ape it was named after. Burger King sells two Whoppers for every one regular hamburger. And the submarine sandwiches at some delis approach arm's length.

Don't buy into all that overeating.

Yeah, we know. It's tough to avoid. Most teens find that it's harder to reduce the amount of food they eat than to eat low-fat food. These tips should help you out:

◆ **Go** fish: Your meat portion—lean meat, fish or poultry—should be 3 to 4 ounces, about the size of a deck of cards.

- **One** potato, 1/2 potato: Your starch intake for the entire day should be one or two slices of bread OR a cup of cooked pasta OR a baked potato (a 3- to 4-ounce tater, not an 8-ounce monster, which you can cut in half).
- Your salad should be a small mound—about two cupped handfuls—not a mountain of mixed greens, tomato, four-leaf clovers, you name it.
- Eat a piece of fruit the size of your fist.
- Two ounces of pretzels—a good amount—will fit into your cupped hand.
- Thumbs up. An ounce of cheese is the size of your thumb.
- Don't fill 'er up. Most people fill up their plates. Simple solution: use a smaller plate, like a salad plate.
- Unstuff yourself. You don't have to clear your plate or eat until you're stuffed. Healthy people never fill up. Save what you don't want for your next meal.
- Buy lunch-size portions of chips or cookies. That way you won't be tempted to rip into more than one single serving.
- Your tip: ______________________________

There you go.

TAKE TEN

Before we say buh-bye (we'll still be in touch, though, at **www.bodypride.com**), we just want to ask that you keep these 10 tips in mind:

1. Practice portion control. Serve up a plate of food, eat it slowly and refrigerate any leftovers right away so you're not tempted to indulge in seconds. (Who wants a second-plate ribbon?)

"I'm in a bowling league and when we go to Vegas it's hard to stay away from the buffets. The main thing I eat are the salads and the chicken, none of the cheeseburgers or desserts. And it's one trip, not two."

---

2. Always exercise. You love it, your body loves it, it's for life. OK? Enough said.

3. Continue to set goals, make plans, take the steps, avoid the potholes, talk nice to yourself and accomplish your dreams using the amazing techniques you've learned in *bodyPRIDE*. Unlike a sitcom, this is not a program that has a beginning and an end.
4. Continue to rely on your family and friends for support. Let them always show you how much you're loved.
5. Hey, don't ignore your DAP. Maybe it won't be a daily thing-to-do anymore, but it'll help any time you're working toward reaching a dream.
6. Continue to eat three meals a day along with a couple of healthy snacks, like fruit. Are we like one of those worn-out dolls where you pull the string and it only repeats one or two things? Yep. Eat three meals. Eat THREE meals. EAT three mEAls....
7. Yikes, here's that broken doll again with the second stuck phrase: Drink your water. Drink YOUR water. DriNK... Uggghhhhhhhh! Make it stop!
8. We won't pull that string anymore if you promise to take your vitamins.
9. Recognize that you know more about what works for your body than anyone else. You know what makes you feel good over the long-term. Plug in to what's good for you, unplug what isn't.
10. Reward yourself for all the good you've accomplished in the last weeks since you first picked up *bodyPRIDE*. You've jumped over the hurdles, avoided the sticky situations, blasted through the mud and have come out clean. Hear the crowds cheering? For the rest of your life, you'll be successful at reaching your dream. Enjoy!

THE END